Dignity Therapy

Final Words for Final Days

Harvey Max Chochinov

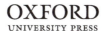

OXFORD
UNIVERSITY PRESS

OXFORD
UNIVERSITY PRESS

Oxford University Press, Inc., publishes works that further Oxford University's objective of excellence in research, scholarship, and education.

Oxford   New York
Auckland   Cape Town   Dar es Salaam   Hong Kong   Karachi
Kuala Lumpur   Madrid   Melbourne   Mexico City   Nairobi
New Delhi   Shanghai   Taipei   Toronto

With offices in
Argentina   Austria   Brazil   Chile   Czech Republic   France   Greece
Guatemala   Hungary   Italy   Japan   Poland   Portugal   Singapore
South Korea   Switzerland   Thailand   Turkey   Ukraine   Vietnam

Copyright © 2012 by Oxford University Press, Inc.

Published by Oxford University Press, Inc.
198 Madison Avenue, New York, New York 10016
www.oup.com

Oxford is a registered trademark of Oxford University Press, Inc.

Library of Congress Cataloging-in-Publication Data

Chochinov, Harvey Max.
Dignity therapy : final words for final days / Harvey Max Chochinov.
p.; cm.
Includes bibliographical references and index.
ISBN 978-0-19-517621-6 (hardcover : alk. paper) 1. Terminally ill—Psychology. 2. Palliative treatment.
3. Terminal care—Psychological aspects. I. Title.
[DNLM: 1. Palliative Care—methods. 2. Terminally Ill—psychology. 3. Personhood. 4. Quality of Life.
5. Right to Die. WB 310]
R726.8C483 2012
616'.029—dc23   2011016652

9 8 7 6 5 4 3 2
Printed in the United States of America on acid-free paper

PREFACE

Jacob, grandson of Abraham and son of Isaac, is the third patriarch of the Jewish people. Toward his final days, as he sensed his own death approaching, he summoned his family to provide them with some final thoughts and reflections. It is hard to imagine how he might have known where to begin. Over the course of his 147 years, he had taken four wives, Rachel, Leah, Bilhah, and Zilpah. Between them, they had borne him thirteen children, with the offspring of his sons destined to become the twelve tribes of Israel, following the Exodus, when the children of Israel settled in the Land of Canaan. As a young man, he had deceived his father and his older brother Esau by receiving the blessing of the first-born. Later, during a vision of a ladder reaching unto heaven, he heard the voice of God and obtained His blessings. While returning to Canaan, hearing that Esau and his army were on their way, he again encountered God, this time in the form of an angel with whom he fought through the night.

Once his family had gathered by his side, history does not record whether Jacob recalled any of these events. What we do know is that he used this occasion to bless his children, each in their own special way. No doubt, his parting words for Reuben, his first born, were tempered by the not so minor issue of incest; Reuben had slept with Bilhad years earlier, and they had never spoken of it, at least not up until now. Between Jacob and his second and third sons, Simeon and Levi, there was the matter of Shechem. To avenge their sister's rape, Simeon and Levi had killed all the men of Shechem, plundered their property, women and children. Jacob did not approve of their actions, and for this reason, saved his primary blessing for his fourth born, Judah. From his eleventh child, Joseph, whom he fathered at the age of 91, Jacob extracted the promise to have his remains placed in the Cave of the Patriarchs with Leah, and Abraham, Sarah, Isaac, and Rebecca. Following his final instructions, Jacob—or as he was then known, Israel—died and soon after, was buried in Canaan.

In Jacob's final words to his family, history records its first *Ethical Will*. Ethical wills, which were initially conveyed orally, were designed as a way of passing traditions and values from one generation to the next. What might Jacob have been feeling over three thousand years ago as he undertook this task? On the one hand, he no doubt saw this as a way to pass along moral values for generations to come.

Perhaps he took some comfort in knowing that, in spite of death, the lessons and insights he most cherished would transcend his departure. In this way, perhaps he felt he was denying death its ability to destroy those parts of him—those beliefs, insights, and lessons—that defined his very essence. There must also have been a feeling, a sense that in spite of his advanced age and fragile health, he was still valued and his life, or whatever little of it that remained, was cherished by those closest to him.

Unlike Jacob, most people have not spoken directly with God, nor taken multiple partners, nor spawned a bevy of children destined to become an entire nation. On the other hand, is it not conceivable that, like Jacob, mere mortals might find comfort in knowing their final thoughts and words are deemed precious; that in spite of illness, they are still valued; and, perhaps, that it is possible to leave something, which will outlive them and be a remembrance to those left behind?

These, of course, are not new ideas. As long as humankind has grappled with mortality, it has found ways to leave behind testimony of its prior existence. Whether one considers prehistoric paintings on cave walls or contemporary monuments that dot the modern landscape, each declares: *"We were here! Don't forget us."* Ways of affirming this declaration are intricately woven into the human drama. A poem, a piece of music, a work of art, an achievement of technological ingenuity—these can outlive their maker, as can the stories each of us has to tell. And might the sharing of these stories provide a source of comfort, for those about to die, as well as those soon to be bereft?

Over the past few decades, the potential for meaning, purpose, and affirmation to assuage suffering has received careful attention in the field of palliative care. Dame Saunders, the founder of the modern hospice movement, said, "You matter because you are you, and you matter to the end of your life."[1] The challenge is how to transform this credo into the delivery of better palliative care. That someone *thinks* you matter *matters naught,* unless they are able to convey that in a way that can readily be perceived and internalized. Jacob's family managed to accomplish this by gathering at his side and taking in his every word, as if each were a precious gem to be held and treasured forever.

Throughout his lifetime, Jacob's inspiration came from heaven above. On the other hand, the inspiration for Dignity Therapy—a novel, individualized psychotherapy targeting people with life-threatening and life-limiting conditions—came from patients taking part in a program of palliative and end-of-life care research.[2-5] While Dignity Therapy may resemble the Ethical Will, life review, personal narrative, or other existential psychotherapies, what differentiates it is its empirical basis. Dignity Therapy can promote spiritual and psychological well-being, engender meaning and hope, and enhance end-of-life experience. It can help people prepare for death and provide comfort in whatever little time they have left. As ephemeral as these outcomes may seem, it is important to recognize that the components of Dignity Therapy, its mode of administration, and the arguments affirming its efficacy—for patients and for their families—are based exclusively on careful, detailed, and novel studies focused on palliative end-of-life care.

Since the conceptual framework underpinning Dignity Therapy was first published in the *Journal of the American Medical Association* in 2002,[6] this therapeutic modality has begun to take hold in many countries around the world. To date, Dignity Therapy has been studied, or is being studied, in Canada, Australia, the United States, China, Japan, Denmark, Sweden, Scotland, Portugal, and England. In addition, Dignity Therapy training workshops have been held in Hong Kong, Taiwan, Argentina, and New Zealand. Despite some minor regional issues and subtle cultural variations, palliative care clinicians worldwide have enthusiastically embraced Dignity Therapy. More important, patients approaching death and their

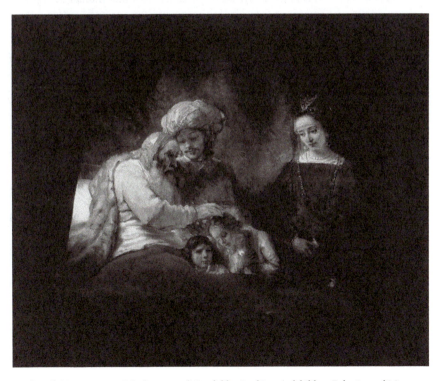

Rembrandt Harmensz van Rijn (1606-1669). Jacob blessing his grandchildren Ephraim and Menasse in the presence of their parents Joseph and Anasth. Canvas.

Photo Credit: Erich Lessing / Art Resource, NY

Germaeldegalerie Alte Meister, Museumslandschaft Hessen Kassel, Kassel, Germany.

families from far and wide have been able to benefit from this brief palliative care psychotherapy.

As with any new treatment, there is tension between wanting to disseminate its use as widely as possible and safeguarding its integrity. Hence, the need for this handbook. *Dignity Therapy: Final Words for Final Days* is the most comprehensive description of Dignity Therapy to date. Readers are offered a detailed accounting of how Dignity Therapy evolved, the current state of evidence supporting its application, and most important, a complete description of how to do Dignity Therapy. Over the years, those of us closely involved with this therapeutic approach have come to respect its potency and its ability to help patients and families from all walks of life and from all regions of the world. We have also come to appreciate that Dignity Therapy, like any other psychotherapy, takes time to master. While this manual will provide you the basics, your therapeutic skill and effectiveness will no doubt evolve over time.

Jacob's final words to his family consisted of sacred blessings and instructions for his burial. Since its inception, Dignity Therapy has been used hundreds if not thousands of times to capture a myriad of circumstances that human beings find themselves in as they exit this world. It is my sincere hope that the practice of Dignity Therapy enriches your work. Most of all, I hope that Dignity Therapy enhances your patients' quality of life and quality of dying, as they confront the inevitability of death.

REFERENCES

1. Saunders C. Care of the dying. 1. The problem of euthanasia. *Nurs Times*. 1976; 72(26): 1003–1005.
2. Chochinov HM, Hack T, McClement S, Kristjanson L, Harlos M. Dignity in the terminally ill: a developing empirical model. *Soc Sci Med*. 2002; 54(3):433–443.
3. Chochinov HM, Hack T, Hassard T, Kristjanson LJ, McClement S, Harlos M. Dignity and psychotherapeutic considerations in end-of-life care. *J Palliat Care*. 2004; 20(3):134–142.
4. McClement SE, Chochinov HM, Hack TF, Kristjanson LJ, Harlos M. Dignity-conserving care: application of research findings to practice. *Int J Palliat Nurs*. 2004; 10(4):173–179.
5. Hack TF, Chochinov HM, Hassard T, Kristjanson LJ, McClement S, & Harlos M. Defining dignity in terminally ill cancer patients: A factor-analytic approach. *PsychoOncology*, 2004; 13:700–708.
6. Chochinov HM. Dignity-conserving care—a new model for palliative care: helping the patient feel valued. *JAMA*. 2002; 287(17):2253–2260.

ACKNOWLEDGMENTS

While dying is inevitable, dying poorly ought not to be. As a psychiatrist and researcher working in palliative care, I am humbled by the capacity of human beings to cope with various painful things, which life invariably brings. I am also humbled by my clinical colleagues' abilities to alleviate pain, lessen suffering, and provide comfort to patients nearing their final days, which is why I think most people have the wrong idea about palliative care. If life is akin to walking a tightrope, the chance of falling increases toward the end. Think then, of palliative care as a safety net. No one escapes falling, but palliative care can provide a softer landing. Those of us who work in this field are focused on how to help patients and families achieve that softer landing. Knowing that it is indeed possible makes this work intriguing, rewarding, and, more than occasionally, awe inspiring.

Of the things I have done in palliative care over the past twenty years, none have been quite as gratifying and personally engaging as Dignity Therapy. Before that work began, my research had examined various dimensions of end-of-life care. Given my training, my natural inclination has been to study the emotional aspects of approaching death. At the outset of my research career, this meant a careful examination of clinical depression in the terminally ill. This led to developing ways to screen for depression, along with studies examining desire for death, will to live, and factors that might influence a patient's wish to go on living in the face of a dire prognosis.

Although this was useful in its own way, it was largely descriptive. In other words, it helped those of us working in palliative care to identify various problems facing dying patients and their families, without necessarily offering any particular solutions (this may be the reason I decided not to become a neurologist; the diagnosis to treatment ratio just seemed too high to be all that much fun). Little did I realize that studying dignity was going to change everything. It is difficult, if not impossible, to respond to problems before being able to clearly articulate what those problems are. The early work on dignity began to identify some of the things that influence a patient's sense of dignity, thus placing those issues on the palliative care radar.

As the work on dignity was coming together, so too was my wonderful research team. One of my dearest friends and colleagues, Dr. Linda Kristjanson, was there from the very outset of the dignity work. Her research skills, integrity, and support have been, and continue to be, a blessing. Dr. Susan McClement is someone that I often refer to as my academic spouse. We share our ideas and work side by side, seeing to it that the research emanating from the Manitoba Palliative Care Research Unit is meaningful and honest. Dr. Thomas Hack has been a core part of our "dignity team" from its very inception; he and I and Sue spent more hours conducting the qualitative data analysis that resulted in the Dignity Model—which forms the basis of Dignity Therapy—than it took to collect the data itself. Dr. Mike Harlos is one of the most talented palliative care clinicians I know. He provides our team an astute clinical eye and a perspective informed by years of providing care to countless patients and their families. Dr. Tom Hassard is our biostatistics maven. His gentle manner, skill, and humanity make him yet another delightful member of our team.

Then there is my team of research nurses. In case anyone has ever wondered why a place like Winnipeg manages to host a successful palliative care research program, the simple answer is this: my research nurses are the best. Katherine Cullihall is compassion personified. She helped me sort through many of the details of the Dignity Therapy protocol as we observed what did and did not work. At this point in time, no one has more experience delivering Dignity Therapy than Katherine. Beverley Cann participated in the randomized control trial of Dignity Therapy. Her combination of honesty and intellect make her an invaluable member of our team; she was also instrumental in organizing and editing this current text. Last but certainly not least is Sheila Lander. Sheila was my very first research nurse and the person who helped gather data for so many of our team's earliest studies. After a brief hiatus, she returned to our team to coordinate the international randomized control trial of Dignity Therapy. As a result, her winning smile and winning ways are now well known and appreciated by my colleagues in New York City and Perth, Australia.

While other members of my team were not directly involved in Dignity Therapy, they deserve mention, as they are part of what makes coming into work each day such a joy. Dr. Nancy McKeen is my research psychologist, and helps ensure that funding keeps coming into the unit to support our work. Miriam Corne is my newest research nurse; if caring came in a bottle, it would surely be called Miriam. Dr. Genevieve Thompson was my postdoctoral student and is now a research associate. Her talent—like her capacity to produce outstanding work—is enormous. Dr. Shane Sinclair is my current postdoctoral student; his enthusiasm and enquiring mind are encouragement to keep looking at the world as a place filled with possibility. Angela Saj is my extraordinary administrative assistant. Without her savvy and guidance, I am convinced nothing would ever get done!

For nearly 25 years, I have been blessed to call Dr. William Breitbart my friend and mentor. In so many ways, Bill is the brother I never had. He was my supervisor when I first came to train at Memorial Sloan-Kettering many years ago. To this day, he can make me laugh like no one else can. Bill and his team took part in the international randomized controlled trial of Dignity Therapy. Other key mentors and supporters along the way include Drs. Jimmie Holland, Keith Wilson, Kathleen Foley, Dhali Dhaliwal, Brent Schacter, William Bebchuk, Samia Barakat, Murray Enns, Brian Postl; Jill Taylor-Brown and John Farber; Senator Sharon Carstairs, Shelly Cory, and Josette Berard.

It is hard to write a book that deals with mortality and the innate vulnerability of human beings without reflecting on my own life. In so many ways, I have been lucky. My parents, Dave and Shirley Chochinov, raised me in a loving and secure home. I married my best friend, Michelle; and our children, Lauren and Rachel, have grown into kind, grounded, intelligent young women. Like most people who have lived into midlife, I have experienced my share of loss. Never to be forgotten include my grandparents, Joseph and Florence Wolodarsky, Max and Pessa Chochinov; my in-laws, Sam and Sheila Sellers and brother-in-law, Shep Nerman; aunts and uncles Jack and Shirley Wolodarsky, Marilyn and Martin Levitt, Fred Lacovetsky, Sid Bagel, Larry Usiskin, Harold Shukster, Norman Chochinov; and my dear sister Ellen Chochinov, to whom this book is dedicated.

Finally, I want to acknowledge the patients and families who took part in Dignity Therapy. Each participated despite profound vulnerability, when time itself was a scarce and ever-decreasing commodity. In doing so, they helped demonstrate how Dignity Therapy can be applied to those whose lives are drawing to a close. I am so grateful for their generosity. I can only hope that they considered having Dignity Therapy a fair exchange for their precious time. You, the reader, are about to hear many of their stories. Determining whether Dignity Therapy might play a role in your practice, and perhaps provide patients nearing death a softer landing, will be for you to decide.

Harvey Max Chochinov
December 12, 2010

CONTENTS

Dignity Therapy

1

DIGNITY AND THE END OF LIFE

The greatest mistake in the treatment of diseases is that there are physicians for the body and physicians for the soul, although the two cannot be separated.

— Plato

WHY STUDY DIGNITY?

Imagine for a moment you are nearing the end of life. There is no way of knowing exactly when this might occur. You could be in the prime of life, when there is still so much to live for, or in your twilight years, after you have had the opportunity to make of your life what you will. Nevertheless, try to imagine what would determine the quality of your remaining days. Perhaps it might be how comfortable you can be made or your sense of personal autonomy. Perhaps the desire to squeeze out life's final drops would depend on the presence of people you love and cherish, and those who love you in return. What would it take, however, to arrive at an impasse when you no longer wished to go on?

Reflection of this sort begins the journey toward understanding dignity-conserving care and the underpinnings of Dignity Therapy. In fact, studies that examined the experience of people who sought help to end their lives provided our first clue to the importance of dignity in patient care. For people considering this stark choice, living, breathing, facing another day might start to feel redundant. Perhaps the most tangible understanding of this choice comes from Holland, where euthanasia and assisted suicide have been practiced for several decades. The Act regulating its practice came into effect in 2002. This Act allows physicians, under certain conditions, to grant the request to hasten death of patients with "unbearable suffering." In order to study the consequences of this legislation, the Dutch government commissioned an examination of the prevalence of Medical Decisions to End Life or MDEL.

The first nationwide Dutch study on euthanasia and other Medical Decisions to End Life (MDEL) consisted of three data sets, including mailed questionnaires to the physicians of 7000 deceased persons, a prospective survey of physicians regarding 2250 deaths, and detailed interviews with 405 physicians who had participated in hastening their patients' deaths by euthanasia or physician-assisted suicide.[1] Alleviation of pain and symptoms with high dosages of opioids that might shorten the patient's life was the most important MDEL, accounting for 17.5% of all deaths. In another 17.5% of patients, death could be ascribed to a non-treatment decision. These were instances when a decision to withhold or to withdraw a treatment no longer deemed to be justified preceded the patient's death. Euthanasia, that is, the administration of lethal drugs at the patient's request, was reported in 1.8% of all deaths. Death from physician-assisted suicide was reported in less than one half of 1%. Another study in 2005 reported that of all deaths in the Netherlands, 1.7% resulted from euthanasia and 0.1% from physician-assisted suicide.[2] The authors speculated that this particular decrease in MDEL might have resulted from the increased use of other end-of-life care interventions such as palliative sedation.

Most health care providers would rather avoid being drawn into conversations about euthanasia and physician-assisted suicide. They assume that a patient's expressed wish to die will force them to walk a dangerous line between not yielding to taking part in a felony on the one hand, while staving off feelings of helplessness and impotence on the other. The legal, moral, and philosophical complexities of these issues are ones that lawyers, ethicists, and policy makers will continue to argue; that said, until quality palliative care is universally available, these arguments may sometimes ring hollow. In the face of an expressed wish to die, however, the role of the health care provider is entirely unique. Clinicians must always try to appreciate the full clinical picture and respond in as therapeutically effective a way as possible. However, to respond empathically to circumstances in which patients have lost their will to live, clinicians need to understand the physical, psychological, spiritual, and existential landscape of the wish to die.

Our research has demonstrated that those who express a wish for an earlier death are more likely to be depressed, experience significant discomfort due to uncontrolled pain, and report less social support.[3] Existential considerations, such as hopelessness, burden to others, and sense of dignity, also have a marked influence on patients' will to live. The Dutch experience, however, offers some important clinical insights, not only about how many patients avail themselves of MDEL, but also why these patients seek out this particular means of ending their lives. Paul van der Maas and his colleagues[1] faced a difficult challenge—the people whose motivation to die was of central interest were no longer alive to share their experiences. To address this rather significant methodological problem, the researchers contacted physicians who had signed death certificates, indicating that the patient had died either as a result of euthanasia or assisted-suicide. While not an ideal research design, under the circumstances, it was likely the best choice available. According to these physicians, "loss of dignity" was the most common reason given for hastening the death of their patient, cited in 57% of cases. Other reasons included pain alone in 5% of cases, pain as part of a constellation of symptoms (46%), being dependent on others (33%), tiredness of life (23%), and unworthy dying (46%).[1]

The reported connection between "sense of dignity" and how it might inform the wish to go on living is as problematic as it is interesting. After all, in the van der Maas study, physicians, rather than patients themselves, were the primary informants describing the role that loss of dignity played in the wish for earlier death. This study raises another question: how does one define a concept as nebulous as "dignity?" Without having given them an a priori definition of how to apply the term dignity to the experiences of their now-deceased patients, physician respondents were left to their own devices, to their own idiosyncratic interpretations of what dignity meant and to determine if, or how, it had been undermined or even violated. These questions were encouragement enough for our research team to launch a new series of investigations; after all, if dignity is worth dying for, surely, it is worth carefully studying.

DIGNITY AND EMPIRICAL RESEARCH

Defending dignity in health care is a bit like defending motherhood and apple pie. At first glance, it might seem unnecessary and perhaps not even worth the bother. After all, dignity, and all that it implies, strikes a chord that resonates with most health care professionals. Like *love* or *joy* or *faith*, one might conclude that *dignity* should be left to intuition and certainly not placed under an empirical lens. While the health care literature is replete with references to dignity as it relates to quality medical care, there is little consistency with how the term is applied. So, for example, people might hold diametrically opposed opinions on various health care practices—euthanasia, assisted suicide, terminal sedation, artificial hydration and nutrition—and ultimately argue that *dignity* is their trump card. Hence, the *right to die* argument may be framed as the ultimate expression of individual autonomy and, therefore, consistent with human dignity, while opponents of this argument see the purposeful taking of human life as an egregious assault on human dignity.

The concept of dignity is afforded a high profile in end-of-life care. Most palliative care providers would agree that dignity is a philosophical cornerstone of their approach to patients and families. However, while patients may be *dying* for lack of dignity, the medical literature is relatively silent on how dying patients experience or understand the notion of dignity—that is, until now. Our first study of dignity took place among patients with end-stage cancer.[4] These patients were registered with one of two urban specialty palliative care units in Winnipeg, Canada: one located in a general hospital, St. Boniface General Hospital, and the other in an extended-care facility, Riverview Health Centre. These units are part of the Winnipeg Regional Health Authority Palliative Care Program, which provides state-of-the-art community-based and inpatient palliative end-of-life care. Patients were not referred to the study if they were cognitively impaired, unable to give informed consent, or simply too unwell to take part in the protocol. Over a four-year period, 213 patients took part, each of whom were asked to rate their sense of dignity. Our main outcome measures included a seven-point sense of dignity scale (0 = no sense of lost dignity, 1 = minimum, 2 = mild, 3 = moderate, 4 = strong, 5 = severe, and 6 = extreme sense of lost dignity); a symptom-distress scale; the McGill pain questionnaire; the index of independence in activities of daily living; a quality-of-life scale; a brief battery of self-report screening measures of desire for death, anxiety, hopelessness, and will to live; burden to others; and ratings of social support.

More than half of all patients reported their sense of dignity as strong or intact, while the remainder indicated that they had at least some, or occasional, dignity-related concerns. Only sixteen patients, or 7.5% of these patients, indicated that loss of dignity was a significant problem, marked by often feeling degraded, ashamed, or embarrassed. These sixteen patients with a fractured sense of dignity were more likely to be hospitalized, as opposed to receiving community-based care, and tended to be younger. Patients with a fractured sense of dignity were more likely to indicate a desire for death or loss of will to live and were also more likely to indicate that they felt depressed, hopeless, or anxious. Not surprising, patients whose dignity was fractured were more likely to report difficulty with bowel functioning and a preoccupation with their appearance. They were also more likely to report a need for help with intimacies of care such as bathing, dressing, or toileting. Overall quality-of-life ratings, and satisfaction with quality of life, were significantly lower in those with a fractured sense of dignity than in those whose dignity was intact. When all of these factors were examined together, a heightened risk for fractured sense of dignity was associated with, in descending order of magnitude, increased perceived change in appearance, increased sense of being a burden to others, increased dependency on others, increased pain intensity, and being an inpatient.[4]

Given that this is one of the first empirical studies to examine the concept of dignity from the perspective of dying patients, a few interpretive observations are warranted. For instance, it was surprising that fewer than 8% of patients in our study reported a significant fractured sense of dignity. When one considers that these patients were all within weeks to a few months of death, a higher incidence of fractured dignity might have been anticipated. Then again, recall that each of these patients was receiving quality, comprehensive, end-of-life care. As with most state-of-the-art programs, the Winnipeg Regional Health Authority Palliative Care Program offers services that address the physical, psychosocial, existential, and spiritual challenges facing patients nearing the end of life. That being the case, the data would suggest that dignity-related concerns are mitigated in circumstances where comprehensive and effective care is provided. Achieving good pain and symptom control, feeling supported, and having personal needs addressed, all decrease the likelihood that dignity will be undermined. A second consideration to explain the relative paucity of dignity-related distress may be how patients view or appreciate their sense of dignity. As one devout elderly woman with an end-stage cancer said, "Dignity is God given . . . as long as I am living, it can't be taken away." In this instance, it is possible to imagine that dignity is aligned with core sense of self or personhood. As such, its resilience would make it impervious to common challenges facing people nearing death.

The prominence of *personal appearance* in association with dignity is quite intriguing. Appearance, or our perception of how we appear to others, is a complex issue. While it can be thought of as internally held, it is also highly dependent on external input; without such validation, it can be difficult to gauge how we are perceived. What then, is the connection between sense of dignity and perceptions of how we are seen?

Many years ago, I saw a young patient with a primary brain tumor. Sadly, his options for cure had long since run out. While many of the details of his case have faded, there is one image that remains especially vivid. One day I arrived at his room to find him moribund. He was no longer able to speak and appeared close to death. As one can imagine, his illness had taken its toll and he was a skeletal remains of the young and healthy person he had once been. This particular morning, someone had placed a picture of him, in a perfect state of health, on his bedside table. I found myself gazing at a photograph of a powerfully built bodybuilder, striking an "incredible hulk like" pose. The contrast between this dying young man and the photograph of the muscular Adonis was jarring. As I left his room, I recall feeling unsettled, trying to sort through the meaning of those two juxtaposed images.

Years later, as the results from our dignity studies accumulated and the issue of appearance and the perception of how we are seen by others began to emerge, the memory of that morning came flooding back, along with a long-belated epiphany: "This is how I need you to see me." Perhaps the discomfort I felt so many years before reflected my own lack of understanding and inability to articulate this message. I was being asked, not to do or say something differently, but rather, to *see* things differently. The photograph, a wordless request, was telling me not to ignore what my eyes were seeing, but rather, to register what my patient was trying to say: "this is who I am;" "this is how I wish you could see me;" "this is how I want to be remembered."

More recent empirical studies on perceptions of dignity have confirmed our initial findings. For example, in a study of 211 patients receiving palliative care, 87.1% said not being treated with respect or understanding and feeling a burden to others were issues most likely to influence their sense of dignity.[5] This should come as little surprise, given that the notion of respect includes the idea of how we are perceived by others. It thus appears, for patients nearing death, that the perception of no longer being treated with respect is highly entangled with the concept of dignity.

THE MODEL OF DIGNITY IN THE TERMINALLY ILL

Dignity is a complex and textured construct; understanding it requires more than merely documenting its association with various end-of-life care issues. Although knowing these connections is both important and interesting, this knowledge falls short of actually describing what dignity is. Saying that dignity correlates with quality of life still falls short of defining dignity. It does not tell us how people with a life-threatening or life-limiting illness experience their sense of dignity; or what things help support, or undermine, a patient's sense of dignity; or whether there are health care provider behaviors that are potent in influencing dignity. Although we may know the prevalence of dignity-related concerns among the dying and the various associations between dignity and common sources of distress, we need a better understanding of how patients appreciate dignity and dignity-related issues as they approach death.

Perhaps the most helpful study, which moved our research group toward those deeper insights, was one we conducted with a cohort of fifty patients who were close to death.[6] Rather than simply rating their sense of dignity, we asked these patients to explain their understanding of dignity in all its complexities. What does dignity mean at this stage in your life? Can you recount instances when your dignity was undermined? Can you remember situations when you felt your dignity was particularly supported? How does your sense of dignity relate to the essence of who you are and the extent to which you experience life as still worth living? What emerged from this detailed inquiry was a first-of-its-kind Model of Dignity in the Terminally Ill (see Figure 1.1).

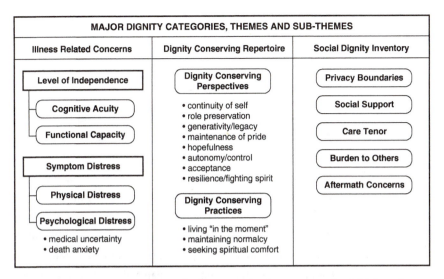

FIG 1.1 **Model of Dignity in the Terminally Ill. Reprinted with permission of** *Social Science &* *Medicine.*

Models, like road maps, can document a complex landscape, guide people on how to get where they need to go, and even occasionally take people to places of which they were entirely unaware. Our Model of Dignity in the Terminally Ill, or simply, the Dignity Model, provides an important overview of how the notion of dignity relates to the broadest range of issues, deemed important by people facing significant, life-threatening, or life-limiting health challenges.

This Dignity Model, based entirely on patient data, indicates there are three primary sources of influence that are of concern to patients. Dignity can be affected by **Illness-Related Concerns**—factors that derive most directly from the illness itself, such as physical and psychological responses. Dignity can also be affected by what we labeled the **Dignity-Conserving Repertoire**. This repertoire describes myriad psychological and spiritual factors that can influence a person's sense of dignity. These factors are often embedded within the patient's psychological makeup, personal background, and accumulated life experiences. Finally, while dignity may be internally mediated, it may also be externally influenced. In other words, there are factors within the social environment that affect a person's sense of dignity. We refer to these external factors or challenges as the **Social Dignity Inventory**.

Illness-Related Concerns

Within the major theme of Illness-Related Concerns, several important subthemes emerge, including level of independence and symptom distress. Level of independence includes the subthemes, cognitive acuity and functional capacity. Symptom distress includes the subthemes, physical distress and psychological distress.

Level of Independence

The way people think about themselves is complex and is based, in part, on the things they are able to do. If one considers the many activities that occupy a normal day, it is easy to see how these meld into one's core sense of self. But is what we do "who we are," or merely the operational functions we carry out? Cleaning the home, preparing a meal, doing the laundry, looking after children, walking the dog, doing the banking, paying bills, driving a car—in the face of no longer being able to do these tasks, what happens to sense of self? At what point do these various functions, alone or cumulatively, conflate with sense of personhood? And what about other activities such as attending a concert, reading a newspaper, devouring a novel, performing in a play, playing an instrument, writing poetry, visiting friends and family, traveling, studying, meditating, exercising—the list is endless. The question is: to what extent do these activities or functions define who we are, how others see us, and how we see ourselves?

Under what circumstances might dependency undermine our core sense of self or personhood? Level of independence conveys the degree to which one is able to avoid feeling reliant on others. For some, accepting help is a necessary and required accommodation, which leaves sense of self unharmed. For others, it is an overwhelming and devastating assault on personhood.

Eric was a twenty-eight-year-old man being treated for testicular cancer. Joan, his wife of two years, was becoming increasingly distressed by the rapid deterioration in their relationship, which seemed to coincide almost exactly with the time that he had been ill. While they had previously gotten along well and, according to Joan, had a solid relationship, everything changed after his diagnosis. Not only were they no longer getting along, but Eric had recently rented and moved into his own apartment. When seen in consultation, what emerged was that he could not stand the idea that he might be seen as anything less than "whole." While he was still basically feeling well, the fact that he could no longer "carry in the groceries," for example, felt shattering and unacceptable to his sense of being a "strong man" and a "good husband."

Two areas that begin to challenge level of independence, and are part of the Dignity Model, include cognitive acuity and functional capacity. The former speaks to one's ability to maintain acute mental processes, without which exercising autonomy becomes more difficult. Fatigue, delirium, primary central nervous system insult, or injury can have a profound impact on level of independence. As discussed later, they can also have a profound impact on sense of self. Little wonder that primary psychotic disorders or the dementias are associated with a high prevalence of clinical depression. In both instances, it is nearly impossible to distance oneself from the implications of illness, given that the target organ is fundamentally *self*. Functional capacity, on the other hand, refers to the ability to carry out various personal tasks such as shopping, cleaning, preparing meals, and the like. The "intimate dependencies", such as eating, bathing, and toileting have been shown to be particularly challenging for patients who express dignity-related concerns. It is important, however, to note that the meaning that patients attach to these activities, and the circumstances in which they occur, have a profound influence on how the patient experiences them.

Joe was a seventy-eight-year-old married gentleman with advanced prostate cancer. While his wife and two adult children were determined to keep him home for his final weeks of life, this was becoming increasingly difficult. During a review of the care plan with the homecare case manager, Joe voiced his wish to be hospitalized. Although it appeared that basic comfort and care were being well managed at home, Joe felt increasingly uncomfortable with his wife having to sometimes "be my nurse." Although she denied any discomfort assisting in tasks such as feeding, bathing, or placing a bedpan, Joe felt shamed. It was not so much that he felt a burden to his wife or that he sensed any resentment or hesitation. Rather, he simply could not accept the dependency he felt so acutely when she had to take on these tasks, and the profound distortion this imposed on their usual role functions. As it turned out, he was hospitalized about a week before he died. He told the nursing staff how much more at peace he felt, knowing that they—and not his family—would be there to attend to this personal care.

People with long-term disabilities provide important insights about the experience of functional dependency.[7] Many disabled individuals require long-term assistance with various activities of daily living, such as dressing, bathing, toileting, or feeding. The dynamics that make this physically, psychologically, and spiritually tenable are enlightening. The care receiver must feel that they are not imposing an unacceptable or unreasonable burden on the carer. Care receivers must feel that getting care is a right and a matter of due course, rather than a favor to be extracted. In some instances, the exchange of a fee, as in the case of a paid caregiver, can render the transaction one that feels equitable and fair. The receiver becomes a consumer of services rather than a cause for charity, pity, or goodwill. The receiver must feel that, in spite of dependency, they are still in charge. Furthermore, they must feel that their specific directions and preferences will determine how things are done and that their "expert opinion" is vital and welcome.

Symptom Distress

Symptom distress is, of course, a profound challenge for those who are ill. Symptoms divert people's attention from other aspects of their life to bodily sensations or concerns. In many instances, symptoms are the doorway to patienthood. Physical distress is always accompanied by myriad feelings and questions. The physical experience of a symptom and its emotional accompaniment are indivisible. For instance, the experience of pain may be accompanied by anxiety, depression, and fear, depending on how the pain is interpreted and what meaning is ascribed to it. These experiences generally reinforce one another. As such, fear or depression tends to make pain less tolerable; conversely, pain can make patients more susceptible to depression or anxiety.

> Mrs. G. was a sixty-four-year-old woman with advanced breast cancer. As her disease progressed, pain control became increasingly problematic. When she developed bone metastasis, her physician recommended that she start on opioid medication. Much to his surprise, however, Mrs. G. outright refused. When seen in consultation, the story emerged that her mother had died about one year before. Just prior to her death, Mrs. G's mother had been started on morphine, became delirious, and in a state of fear and confusion, died shortly thereafter. For Mrs. G., accepting analgesics that included opioids invariably meant that she would follow her mother's unhappy course. Once she was able to articulate this, and disentangle her own circumstances from those of her mother, she was willing to accept analgesia and her pain was quickly controlled. At her follow-up outpatient appointment, now pain free, she spoke of the simple pleasures she was again able to enjoy, including sitting on her backyard patio, drinking a cup of coffee, reading the paper, and feeling the sunshine on her back.

Psychological distress is so profoundly entwined within patienthood. Depression, anxiety, and fear are all ways in which we respond to changing health circumstances, whether actual or threatened. It is noteworthy that medical uncertainty and death anxiety emerge as separate subthemes within psychological distress in the Dignity Model.[6,8] Medical uncertainty is the equivalent of traveling in the dark; without light, the course appears all the more ominous and frightening. Often, patients fear what they don't know, as much, if not more than, what they do know.

The confirmation, even of a serious diagnosis, can provide comfort for someone who has been living with uncertainty, while trying to interpret mounting discomfort or increasing disability. Fear, based on *not knowing*, can segue to finding ways to face what lies ahead, devising coping strategies, or identifying options that might still be viable.

As peculiar and macabre as it sounds, not knowing how death will arrive or be experienced—death anxiety[9,10]—can often be quelled by clear information accompanied by assurances about how distress or problems will be managed and reassurance that the patient will *never* be abandoned. For instance, patients may worry that their analgesics will wear off and that their final days of life will be fraught with terrible pain. Other patients may fear that their breathing will worsen and that they will experience death as a slow suffocation. Others may be concerned that their mental status will change and that they may say or do things that would cause them embarrassment or shame. In every instance, it is possible to allay these fears by providing assurances that these problems can be anticipated and averted by vigilant and effective care. Like walking a high tightrope, the journey is profoundly shaped by the certainty that a safety net awaits below.

Dignity-Conserving Repertoire

Bear in mind that the way someone responds to illness is not determined solely by the illness, but by the entirety of who they are. Every person has a particular psychological makeup and spiritual outlook that shapes his or her worldview and response to opportunities and crises. In the Model of Dignity in the Terminally Ill, this phenomenon is referred to as the Dignity-Conserving Repertoire.[6,8] The various components of this repertoire provide a framework for understanding how people react to changing health care circumstances.

> A gentle, soft-spoken, elderly physician, just presented with results confirming his malignant brain tumor, responded in true form by uttering "well, this is annoying." A self-loathing young woman, whose childhood was marred by neglect and abuse, experienced a recent diagnosis of ovarian cancer as affirmation of her lack of worth and deservedness of punishment.

Although it is important to understand a patient's response in the here and now, a fuller appreciation for what they might be feeling can only be gleaned through an appreciation of their Dignity-Conserving Repertoire. The Dignity-Conserving Repertoire consists of dignity-conserving perspectives and dignity-conserving practices.

Dignity-Conserving Perspectives

Dignity-conserving perspectives refers to an outlook, or a way of seeing the world, that is dominated, or shaped, by *who* is ill rather than simply by *what* ails them. Everyone has his or her own way of facing, or not facing, adverse life events or circumstances. The psychological or spiritual landscape on which this reaction is played out is referred to as dignity-conserving perspectives. There are eight specific subthemes that describe these perspectives: continuity of self, role preservation, generativity or legacy, maintenance of pride, hopefulness, autonomy or control, acceptance, and resilience or fighting spirit.

Continuity of self. Am I still me? It may seem an odd question, but for someone facing serious illness and mounting losses, it is a question of profound significance. Challenges to continuity of self begin upon entry to patienthood. They can be subtle and, if time-limited, barely noticeable: adjusting one's schedule for a medical appointment, wearing an identification bracelet or hospital-issue clothing, being examined by health professionals, submitting to various tests. The very act of revealing a symptom to a health care provider can alter ones sense of personhood. For a moment in time, be it a breast lump, rectal bleeding, a swollen ankle, a sore throat—at that instant, it is that lump, that rectum, that ankle, that throat that fully occupies the professional's critical gaze.

> A young woman being treated for a benign rectal cyst, after weeks of daily dressing changes by various homecare nurses, lamented that so many people had seen her backside, she felt without dignity: "my doctor probably doesn't even know what my face looks like!"

Like this woman, many patients bemoan the fact that illness can strip them, not just of clothing and modesty, but also of their identity. In spite of the various and complex roles that people play in life, the accomplishments they take pride in, the challenges they face, their hopes, dreams, or fantasies, all can quickly be eclipsed by a symptom or constellation of symptoms that bring them to medical attention.

Continuity of self speaks to the extent that patients are able to maintain their sense of self or personhood, in spite of changing health circumstances. Of course, this will be influenced by a multitude of factors, including the person's psychological makeup, social network, and spiritual or existential outlook. It is the resilience and admixture of these that will determine a person's ability to maintain a sense of identity beyond that of being a patient.

> Mary was a thirty-six-year-old woman with leukemia who required a bone marrow transplant. Almost from the moment of being admitted to the ward, she

found the adjustments to "patienthood" intolerable. The ward routines, her limited mobility because of low blood counts, the innumerable health care workers assigned to various highly specialized aspects of her care—all left her feeling overwhelmed. One day, Mary emerged from her room wearing a long, elegant, blue satin nightgown. While some staff members assumed that this was an expression of little more than vanity, to Mary, it was a way of being able to assert her individuality, even in the face of a life-threatening illness.

Although continuity of self is pertinent to everyone who confronts patienthood, it becomes especially profound for patients facing life-threatening or life-limiting conditions. The illness itself can cause mounting disability and various limitations as part of a downward spiral of diminished functional capacity. While "who we are" may not be the same as "what we do," the two obviously overlap. What happens to personhood when illness disrupts the ability to perform usual activities? For example, a successful research scientist who suffered a stroke was faced with the realization that he could no longer pursue his previous career path, nor could he maintain his intense involvement in student education. While he needed to adjust to diminished vision and reduced hearing, the most profound challenges were of an existential nature: Who am I? What's to become of me? Does my life now have any real value or serve any particular purpose?

Role preservation. To fend off an assault on identity due to illness, patients do their utmost to cling to important, previously held, roles. These roles, and their associated responsibilities, are the bricks and mortar of self; so long as they are intact, the walls of identity hold strong. The closer a threatened role is identified with core self, the greater the risk to personhood. I recall a classical violinist whose entire world revolved around his ability to perform. When he could no longer play due to complications of his treatment for head and neck cancer, in spite of a reasonably good prognosis, he pronounced, "The doctors tell me I should be able to have a reasonable quality of life . . . what life?"

As we move through successive stages of the human life cycle, each of us accumulates many roles and responsibilities. Illness can whittle away at these, sometimes at the margins, and in other instances, at the very core of self. Maintaining roles or some semblance thereof—in spite of fear, fatigue, or discomfort—can be a way of staving off the existential consequences of being ill. Going into the office may not just be a manifestation of commitment to a business or vocational venture but also a psychological strategy to fend off a sense of disintegrating self.

The challenge for patients is to accommodate minor losses while finding ways to safeguard against more serious assaults on personhood. For example, the devoted homemaker and mother who can no longer independently shop for groceries or manage household routines may have to learn to accept assistance, such as being accompanied by a friend or family member and perhaps using a walker or wheelchair to maintain her mobility. Should functional capacity continue to deteriorate, she may no longer be able to shop at all but perhaps may still be involved in preparing meals. When that is no longer possible, role preservation may take the form of helping her family plan menus or instructing them on how her recipes are organized and where they are stored. Each incremental loss of functional independence is associated with having to locate a sense of self that is least encumbered by the illness, where one can try to maintain core critical identities. This inward retreat is driven by loss of functional capacity, whereby previously held roles are relinquished in the service of maintaining those closest to the core. "I may not be able to shop or prepare meals, but I can still nurture my family." In this instance, even the complete relinquishment of a previously held role is offset by safeguarding the symbolic significance of what that role stood for or accomplished. Such accommodation and refinement of how one perceives and enacts previously held roles allows patients to maintain or extend their sense of self and purpose in the face of various losses that illness will invariable claim.

Generativity or legacy. Erik Erikson, a developmental psychologist, believed that "human personality, in principle, develops according to steps predetermined in the growing person's readiness to be driven toward, to be aware of, and to interact with a widening social radius."[11] In middle adulthood, he believed, people enter into a stage of development that he called "Generativity versus Stagnation." *Generativity* refers to providing guidance for the next generation, and it becomes paramount when patients are facing a life-threatening or life-limiting prognosis. In those circumstances, generativity often finds patients contemplating how to extend their influence beyond death itself. Existential confrontation with approaching death raises many questions: What is the meaning of my existence? What has my life amounted to? And, as pressing a concern: Once I am gone, what difference will my life have made?

People deal with this issue in a variety of ways. One aging grandmother, whose daughter was "expecting," felt she was not likely to live long enough for this grandchild to establish any real or lasting memory of her. She decided to write a series of letters to her unborn grandchild, which could be passed along when her parents felt appropriate. Undertaking this project renewed this grandmother's sense of meaning and purpose in life and made her feel that her thoughts, memories, advice, and words of love would live beyond her.

The concept of generativity or legacy is highly pertinent to the underpinnings of Dignity Therapy. Participants who take part in Dignity Therapy are invited to speak about important aspects of their life—things they would want others to know or remember. A carefully constructed framework of questions guides participants to share their thoughts, reminiscences, advice, hopes, and dreams with those they are about to leave behind. These conversations are audio-recorded, transcribed, edited, and returned to the participant so that he or she may share the contents of the document with loved ones.

Dignity Therapy participants have used this generativity exercise in various and creative ways. One sixty-year-old single mother with advanced ovarian cancer used Dignity Therapy as an opportunity to record her life accomplishments for her children and grandchildren, along with providing them instruction on how to incorporate a deeper religious commitment into their daily lives. An aging man with alcoholism and end-stage prostate cancer used this as an occasion to warn his grandchildren not to follow the pattern of his life, and not to squander precious opportunities that might come their way. One young woman dying of breast cancer used Dignity Therapy as a way of sharing with her young daughter the derivation of her daughter's name. A middle-aged businessman, facing a dire prognosis with metastatic lung cancer, used Dignity Therapy to leave behind instructions for his teen-aged children ("be happy, don't forget to exercise, and it might be a good idea to lose some weight"). Within his Dignity Therapy, he also gave his wife explicit permission to remarry, should she find someone to share her life with after his death. More about Dignity Therapy in later chapters.

Maintenance of pride. If experiencing illness can undermine a person's sense of self, then maintaining pride can be understood as a defensive, or coping, strategy to stave off the psychological and existential impact of these assaults. In essence, pride refers to a patient's ability to maintain positive self-regard or self-respect. Illness or symptoms tend to divert attention away from "who I am" and redirect it to "what I have." While stepping into patienthood carries the risk of becoming identified with a particular ailment, maintaining pride helps patients safeguard their sense of personhood.

What we take pride in generally reflects the image we want others to see or to know us by. This may take the form of accomplishments, titles, history, worldview, personal style, special attributes, talents, or skills. These are characteristics that distinguish us from others and make us who we are or, more precisely, how we want to be seen or known. As sickness mounts, so too does vulnerability; sensitivity to assaults on self can become more pronounced. In these instances, even subtleties can have a major impact. An elderly woman receiving hospice care, for example, felt deeply offended that a young physician would presume to address her by her first name. With illness laying claim to so much, such a seemingly innocent presumption can further challenge an already fragile sense of self.

Patients demonstrate various ways of maintaining pride. Subtle assertions of pride may be expressed in how patients choose to be addressed or the placement of a photograph on a bedside table. Sometimes, affirmation of pride can be seen in how patients dress or the people they have accompany them to appointments. A measure of pride can be inferred in how deferential or assertive patients are with health care staff. Sometimes, maintaining pride can be achieved more explicitly. Given the opportunity, patients will share their stories, or at least those details that they believe need to be heard in order to feel acknowledged. This might include some mention of their vocation, family, passions, or interests—in essence, the things without which they might feel naked, vulnerable, and anonymous.

An elderly man, having suffered a series of small strokes, had been hospitalized for the treatment of a stubborn bronchial infection. When seen on morning ward rounds, he was no longer able to speak but was nevertheless cooperative. At the completion of his examination, the attending physician suggested that this would be a good opportunity to have his five medical students and junior resident practice doing rectal examinations. Although he passively submitted, it was unclear how well the patient understood what he was consenting to. I was the last of those students and I cannot, or perhaps do not want to, recall if I performed the examination. What I do remember are the few tears I saw rolling down the patient's face as I exited his room.

Clearly, without some acknowledgment of who they are and sensitivity regarding how they might feel, patients may deem themselves little more than their ailment and defenseless in the face of the perceived objectivity and indifference of health care providers.

Hopefulness. The notion of hope or hopefulness is a moving target in the context of changing health circumstances. Under normal conditions, the idea of hope is connected to one's future expectations and predicated on the assumption that there will be a future. As illness imposes itself, hope must be reconciled between what the disease may claim and what time may still have to offer.[12,13] In these circumstances, hope is typically anticipating a favorable prognosis, a robust treatment response, or a meaningful, protracted reprieve. Taking this to its natural conclusion, it might be expected that overwhelming illness, *de facto,* would obliterate hope. Such, however, is not the case.

As counterintuitive at it might seem, only a minority of terminally ill patients exhibit marked hopelessness. And yet, how can this be, in the face of a prognosis that is indeed hopeless? Clearly, the meaning of hope shifts as curative possibilities begin to fade. Rather than being predicated on time, hope, toward the end of life, is intimately connected to notions of meaning and purpose. Without such hope, loss of the will to live or a heightened desire for death is much more likely.

In a study of 196 patients with advanced terminal cancer, we used a semistructured interview to assess hopelessness and suicidal ideation, along with applying a standard measure for depressive symptoms. We found that hopelessness correlated more highly with suicidal ideation than the level of depression and that hopelessness is a potent predictor of suicidal thoughts, over and above the influence of depression. For health care providers attending to the needs of dying patients, the message is clear: hopelessness is an important clinical marker of suicidal ideation in this vulnerable patient population.[14]

Mr. G. was a sixty-eight-year-old married gentleman with an end-stage gastrointestinal malignancy. He had recently decided that, in view of his illness and the inability to do the things he had formerly loved, he would rather die quickly. To encourage this outcome, he had gone on a hunger strike, resulting in his admission to hospital. As part of a thorough evaluation, I was asked to see him for a psychiatric consultation. He expressed a wish to die, or as he put it, "to press the button right now." Given that he did not meet criteria for major depression or any other overt psychiatric disorder, he was not offered psychopharmaceuticals. He was, however, offered the opportunity to take part in Dignity Therapy. It was explained that this would involve his being able to record his thoughts and feelings for the benefit of his surviving family members, including his wife and several children. Before leaving him, and having made arrangements to return the following day to make the recording, I asked Mr. G. if he would still wish to "push the button now." He responded, "No, I'd like to do this first."

Thus it appears that an effective antidote to hopelessness is reconnecting patients with something that may provide them a continued sense of meaning and purpose.

Autonomy/Control. The extent to which one is able to carry out various functions reflects personal autonomy or control. Unlike level of independence, autonomy/ control is internally mediated; that is, it depends more on one's state of mind than the state of one's body or ability to carry out tasks independently. For example, the patient who, in spite of paralysis, is able to direct her own care or make medical decisions demonstrates a considerable level of autonomy/control. The elderly, stern matriarch, who as her daughter described it, "with a wave of her finger [from her hospice bed], was still in charge" and able to make the rest of her family "jump," maintained her autonomy/control, almost to her final breath.

If autonomy and control are not wholly reliant on level of independence or functional capacity, can they be maintained in the face of utter dependency? The story of the French journalist and author Jean Dominique Bauby provides an affirmative and poignant answer. Bauby was the former editor of *Elle Magazine*, a women's high-fashion journal. On December 8, 1995, at the age of forty-three, he suffered a massive stroke, causing what neurologists refer to as locked-in syndrome. This is a neurological catastrophe, marked by complete paralysis and the inability to communicate with the outside world—despite being cognitively intact, the patient, in essence, is locked inside his or her body. After twenty days in a coma, he awoke to find himself mute and paralyzed. He could, however, move his head a little, produce guttural noises, and blink his left eyelid.

Working with a speech therapist, a coding system was devised wherein the most frequent letter in the French alphabet corresponded to one blink of an eye, the second most frequent letter to two blinks of an eye, and so forth. In this way, Bauby was able to "blink-out" his memoir—*The Diving Bell and the Butterfly*.[15] Because of his condition, he had to compose and edit the book entirely in his head. As the title suggests, the book is metaphorically about a man trapped inside of the dead weight of a diving bell (scuba-like gear) and the places his mind, with the ease of a butterfly, is able to take him. By way of imagination and memory, he is able to share special moments from his past, provide a glimpse of his rich fantasy life, offer reflections on his changed health circumstances, and describe his reactions to his sometimes oblivious caregivers. The book was published in France on March 6, 1997 and was greeted by nationwide accolades. Bauby died three days later due to heart failure.

While Bauby's writing is marvelous and his stories poignant without being maudlin, what is most remarkable about his book is the fact that his words stand as testimony to his post-stroke existence. It is as if someone has fallen into a deep, dark well; it is easy to assume that he has vanished, that he no longer exists, that he could not possibly have survived the fall. Then you hear a voice and realize that, although he is out of sight, he is miraculously alive. Can you imagine the shock of his family, his doctors, the nurses and health care aids when they realized that, buried inside of this seemingly inert body, Bauby had survived the fall? With every grunt, every gesticulation, and finally through the eloquence of his words, Bauby was able to affirm: "I exist; I am still me."

> Today is Father's Day. Until my stroke, we had felt no need to fit this made-up holiday into our emotional calendar. But today we spend the whole of the symbolic day together, affirming that even a rough sketch, a shadow, a tiny fragment of a dad is still a dad.[15]

Exercising autonomy is tangible evidence of one's continued existence. As Bauby himself put it, "If I must drool, I may as well drool on cashmere." In finding the strength and courage to make his voice heard, Bauby taught us the resilience of autonomy, and how its survival has as much to do with mental and spiritual fortitude as retained physical capacity.

Acceptance. Within the Dignity Model, *acceptance* speaks of the ability to adapt to changing health circumstances. It is very clear that as life progresses, people change, as do their attitudes and outlooks. What seems important in youth may no longer feel so pressing as we grow older. As the years pass, dependency, a sense of frailty, or health ailments that would have one time felt unimaginable and totally unacceptable become annoyances that must be accommodated. In our studies, we have found that younger patients, more so than seniors, are more likely to report that inability to carry out tasks of daily living, problems attending to bodily functions, thoughts about how life might end, concerns related to sense of privacy, and difficulty with acceptance can undermine sense of dignity.[16] It would appear that in general, older patients have had more time to experience, learn from, and adjust to the vagaries of life, be they the need to accept help, accommodate to dependency, or confront vulnerability and life's uncertainties. At the same time, age and experience bring the realization that certain things are beyond our control and that life can be as unpredictable and indiscriminant in bestowing its blessings as it is in assigning calamities. There is no explanation for why a twenty-nine-year-old, recently married woman with young children finds herself facing a diagnosis of cancer, while her 89-year-old grandmother continues to participate in community activities, swims four times weekly at a local pool, and has little more than arthritic pain that gets somewhat worse with the cold or damp weather. None of us know what tomorrow brings, aside from an ever-growing awareness that we, too, are vulnerable and life is fragile and finite.

Acceptance is sometimes misconstrued as the need to "be at peace," whatever the health circumstances happen to be. Palliative care, for example, does itself a disservice when some of its practitioners feel that in order to do right by their patients, "death talk" needs to be served up as frequently as meals or analgesia. Acceptance is about making gradual adjustments to changing life circumstances, ideally at a pace that can be tolerated. So long as it does not interfere with care, denial can provide patients the psychological space they need, allowing the reality of their deteriorating health to penetrate gradually, in more manageable increments. Acceptance often comes in small gradations approaching the insight required to make informed decisions about life and treatment.

Anna was a twenty-seven-year-old, recently married woman with stage IV breast cancer. She was also her parents' only child. As her medical circumstances worsened and the *imminence* of her death became evident, the health care staff found themselves struggling with how to address some of the difficult issues that needed to be broached. This was particularly challenging, given Anna's own apparent reticence to talk about things that she found too upsetting. While everyone agreed, for example, that cardiopulmonary resuscitation would essentially amount to little more than a futile assault, conversations about code status had still not taken place.

I was introduced to Anna with the hope that we might be able to make some headway in clarifying what she knew, what she wanted to know, and what decisions she might want to make or have made on her behalf. For the first session or two, we got to know one another and established a comfortable and safe space to talk. About the third session, she used the term "the scary stuff" in reference to those things she knew she was working hard to suppress. Sometimes this "scary stuff" appeared in her dreams and sometimes she felt it dragging her, like a rip-tide, into water beyond her depth. Without ever using the words "death" or "dying," we established that if her heart and lungs stopped working, she would not want them to be kept going artificially. Careful attention to her language and the subtle openings she provided allowed Anna to convey her feelings, thoughts, and wishes to the people she loved and who, in her own way, she sensed would soon be leaving behind.

Resilience and fighting spirit. At its most basic, resilience consists of having the internal strength or fortitude to face whatever lies ahead. For some, this means holding onto the hope of a life-prolonging outcome, while for others, time-limited goals can provide the encouragement needed to carry on. This type of fighting spirit can be a double-edged sword. Although positive thinking can give patients a sense of being in control, it sometimes does so by making them feel responsible for how the course of their disease unfolds. Failure to improve or, worse yet, continuing to decline can be perceived as a personal failure, weakness, or a lack of mental resolve to stave off the unyielding assault of declining health. For others, resilience is more about equanimity, that is, feeling that there is a psychological or spiritual safety net that will provide for a gentle landing, no matter what the outcome. The perceived reliability and strength of this safety net varies from person to person. While one patient may appear to crumble in response to a perceived threat, another seems to find strength in the face of changing health circumstances.

To complicate things further, it takes strength to allow illness to penetrate one's psychological defenses and thus to encounter the uncertainty, pain, and vulnerability of an unknowable future. When "strength" is portrayed as unwillingness or inability to allow the vagaries of illness to penetrate consciousness, it often betrays a weak psychological position. One of our studies found that terminally ill patients who maintain a complete disavowal of their prognosis are more likely to be suffering underlying depression.[17] Resilience, like time, rarely stands still. It can fluctuate concurrently with the disease course itself and is further shaped by the nature of one's support network, belief system, and the ability to ascribe meaning or purpose to one's very existence.

Joan was a fifty-eight-year-old retired nurse in her final stage of metastatic breast cancer. Never married, her closest relationships were with her sister, brother-in-law, and their two daughters. During a visit we had in the palliative care unit, she spoke about her life, her career, and her loving nieces. Joan was a woman of deep religious faith. She described her connection with G-d as feeling, not so much like a shield, but rather, a comforting omnipresence. She became tearful when asked about her fears, admitting she was worried about indignities she might suffer when no longer able to fend for herself. She took comfort in the thought that as she departed this world, the Hand of G-d would take her own hand, and she would not feel alone.

Dignity-Conserving Practices

Dignity-conserving practices are behaviors or activities that enable someone to deal with his or her changing life circumstances.

A forty-year-old single woman with stage IV breast cancer was referred to a group psychotherapy trial designed for women with advanced disease. From the outset, she found it hard to engage in group therapy, marked by a reluctance to get too close to any of the group members. Overall, she felt that the sessions left her feeling depleted and more frightened than ever and worked against her inclination to fight being identified as a "cancer patient." After a few sessions, she decided that heading to Europe and "finding a French lover" was going to do her more good than attending group. Immersing herself in living out this particular fantasy, at least for the moment, suited her better than continuing in therapy.

Living in the moment. The nature of life-threatening or life-limiting illness is that it tends to cast the mind forward. The word *prognosis* derives from the Greek *prógnōsis*, meaning "advanced knowledge,"[18] and attests to how illness forces the mind into the future, toward advanced knowledge that can be anticipated but never fully known. This kind of looking ahead is innately human. Yet the more we do so, the less we are able to focus on our immediate surroundings, thus rendering us frightened and less engaged in the present.

Living in the moment is what people do when they are able to stop themselves from what can turn into overwhelming "forward thinking." Taking in the *here and now* can provide tremendous comfort, offering moments of human contact, love, celebration, humor, affirmation, and, on occasion, even reconciliation. Despite a limited prognosis, people are disinclined to constantly stare that particular reality in the face. Living in the moment is a comforting form of engagement, and it is this very engagement that can transform the final phase of life into a time of living, rather than simply a time of anticipating death.

The process of dying has its own natural way of imposing disengagement by way of overwhelming fatigue, depletion of energy, fewer periods of wakefulness, and eventually, the relinquishing of consciousness itself. But until then, opportunities for moments of engagement can occur, and those moments—whether banal, profound or, most often, somewhere in between—constitute the nature of life's final chapter.

An afternoon on a palliative care unit brings memories of a multitude of such moments of engagement.

An elderly aboriginal woman, enjoying a pleasant visit with her son, tells me about her upbringing and the joys of seeing her children making good lives for themselves and their families.

A husband and wife work out how he will manage to get around in anticipation of being discharged home later that day. She describes him as a neighborhood handyman; he takes pride in describing his various talents, ranging from plumbing to carpentry and auto repair.

A brother and his wife are spending a pleasant afternoon visiting his sister with advanced cancer. Until my arrival, they have been discussing their children and what each is planning on doing the following academic year. Her sister-in-law begins to tell me about my patient's talent as an artist, following which my patient describes a few of her most cherished paintings and who she hopes will eventually have them. Although at one point she mentions occasionally feeling fearful and hopes she will find comfort in her faith "when the time comes," it is the only mention of death I recall hearing over the course of that particular afternoon.

Maintaining normalcy. For each of us, much of day-to-day life falls into various patterns and routines. Not that any two days are exactly alike, but there are similarities that are highly predictable and easily recognized—washing and dressing in the morning, reading a daily paper, watching a regular television show, exercise, cooking, reading, playing music, working at the office, helping children with homework. The list of activities is as variable as are the people who incorporate them into the patterns of their lives. While operationally, many of these may seem rather trite or unimportant, within the psychological and existential realm, they can be highly meaningful. Maintaining usual routines and living day to day—as long, and to the extent, possible—are ways of clinging to the familiar and, therefore, not relinquishing what we know and, ultimately, who we are.

An elderly lawyer with advanced cancer insisted, despite the protestations of his family, on driving into the office each day. While he was no longer well enough to see clients, he maintained that he was well enough to sort through various papers and participate in legal discussions with junior and senior colleagues. When he was no longer well enough to drive, he arranged rides to and from the office, albeit only for a few hours any given day. His family continued to pressure him to stop, as they felt he was pushing himself too hard and that he was taking on tasks that were likely to add to his burden of distress and responsibilities. Finally, when this came to a confrontation with his family—particularly his wife—he was able to explain that the routine of going to the office offered him a reprieve from a "full-time vocation of being a patient." Although he recognized that his office days were numbered, maintaining that contact, for now, provided a well-honed routine, which he saw as a small sanctuary of normalcy.

Seeking spiritual comfort. Like dignity, the term *spirituality* carries different meanings for people as they draw closer to death. For some, spirituality is synonymous with religiosity, with enquiries about spiritual well-being and spiritual support easily moving into discussions about a higher power or Deity, life after death, or one's connections with members or leaders of a particular religious community. In these instances, the language of spirituality readily and comfortably embraces a more formal religious lexicon, opening up various possibilities for providing comfort and support to patients and families who are so inclined.

In my experience, religious convictions do not necessarily lead to specific or predictable modes of end-of-life coping. Two highly contrasting examples illustrate this point. In one instance, a nun in her mid-sixties, a member of a local religious order, was nearing the end of her treatment options for leukemia. In spite of being fully aware of her dire prognosis and knowing that death was imminent, she seemed entirely accepting of her fate and quite at peace. She expressed deep faith and absolute conviction that her future was entirely in God's hands. The memory of her peaceful countenance, magnanimity, and grace is one that has lingered, all of these years later.

The other case is one of a rabbi in his early seventies, who was dying of a primary brain tumor. Over the course of his lifetime, he had dedicated himself to his religious community and adhered faithfully to his religious convictions. He was a Holocaust survivor and had lost many members of his family to Nazi atrocities. Toward the end of his illness, he started to recall many of the horrific memories of his internment and began to think of the consequences of his cancer as a revictimization. His stalwart faith, which had so long defined the essence of who he was, began to waver in the months preceding his death. He had somehow expected that a lifetime of devotion would protect him from what he felt was an unjust and cruel fate. Disappointment and fear found him questioning the benevolence of God and the injustice of His plans for His long faithful servant.

For many people, spirituality is understood, experienced, and practiced in nonreligious ways. Although they may not belief in a deity, higher power, or supreme being, individuals who describe themselves as spiritual often feel a sense of connectedness to things beyond themselves, such as nature, ideas, the human collective, or even time itself. And although this spirituality can be hard to describe, varying as it does from one person to the next, it often contains a quality of inspiration, mystery, or transcendence that imbues life with an overarching sense of meaning and purpose. These two aspects of spirituality, a religious dimension and a meaning and purpose dimension, have been examined by our research group to discern their influence on various facets of end-of-life coping. We have found that feeling one's life has enduring meaning and purpose seems to buffer patients from various kinds of end-of-life distress, including psychological (e.g. anxiety, depression, uncertainty), physical (e.g. not being able to attend to bodily functions, experiencing physically distressing symptoms) and existential (e.g. "no longer feeling like who I was," feelings of unfinished business, not feeling worthwhile or valued) sources of suffering.[16]

Perhaps the biggest challenge in addressing spiritual care for dying patients is presented by those who express no sense of spirituality whatsoever. In such instances, the primary obstacle is often language. As in all facets of palliative care, words are powerful and, depending on how we use them, can soothe, harm, or alienate. Asked the question, "are there spiritual concerns that you might like help with?" the ardent secularist might respond through a filter of utter disconnection, equivalent to being addressed in a foreign language or offered a selection of unfamiliar and unwanted delicacies. Patients reacting this way may conflate the term *spirituality* with *religiosity*, leaving them feeling, at best, misunderstood ("I'm just not inclined that way") or, at worst, offended or alienated. Therefore, clinicians wanting to inquire about spirituality need to choose their words with sensitivity. Avoid making assumptions and provide an entrée that is as wide and accessible as possible. For instance, asking, "Are there things at this time that give life particular meaning or purpose?" is probably open-ended enough to broach a spiritual dialogue without alienating anyone. After such an opening, clinicians must pay careful attention to the patient's leads and choice of words. In some instances, the conversation will stay in a secular realm; at other times, it may move into a more religious sphere. Achieving the right linguistic tone can help patients discover a comfort zone wherein language resonates with their own particular view and orientation toward spirituality and its place within their lives.

Social Dignity Inventory

The defining characteristic of the Social Dignity Inventory is its reference to social issues or relationship dynamics that enhance or detract from a patient's sense of dignity. Dignity is often conceived as having intrinsic and extrinsic components. Illness-Related Concerns and the Dignity-Conserving Repertoire would be subsumed under the former; hence, delineating internalized physical, psychological, and existential factors that influence one's sense of dignity. The Social Dignity Inventory, which conceptually overlaps with the extrinsic components of dignity, refers to how other people and environmental circumstances can influence a patient's sense of dignity.[6,8] It is worth underscoring that the word *dignity* means "to be worthy of honor, respect, or esteem." Besides considering oneself worthy, are those messages of worthiness being externally conferred or validated? Because the Social Dignity Inventory implicates others in the mediation of dignity, it is especially important in terms of how family, friends, and, of course, health care providers interact with and behave toward people nearing the end of life. There are five elements within the Social Dignity Inventory: privacy boundaries, social support, care tenor, burden to others and aftermath concerns.

Privacy Boundaries

Illness lays claim to many things, and privacy is among its first casualties. From the moment we suspect something is wrong with our bodies or how they function, privacy begins to wane. Exposure to examination is only a beginning, with graver illness heralding more ubiquitous privacy disruptions. For patients nearing the end of life, assistance with bathing, dressing, and toileting—what we refer to as the *intimate dependencies*—often become part of routine care. Compassionate caregivers must always be mindful that for the person receiving this kind of assistance, there is nothing routine whatsoever about these necessary, albeit profound compromises to privacy.

Serious illness frequently challenges other aspects of privacy, pushing these boundaries in various ways. To remain in their homes, patients must often rely on various forms of assistance to forestall some form of institutional care. When patients must depend on family, sacrifices of privacy may be compounded by a sense of role disruption or altered sense of self. When children or partners become caregivers, not only is privacy challenged, but, more profoundly, so too is a sense of world order. This is not to say that these transitions cannot be negotiated, but that doing so requires being attentive to the physical, as well as existential demands.

Being healthy allows people to continuously manage the balance between social contact and privacy, usually quite independently and with relative ease. Illness disrupts these delicate modulations, both by virtue of limited energy, as well as through various interruptions over which patients have little influence, such as health care visits, home care schedules, and unanticipated visitors. Most health care settings are also associated with many disruptions that punctuate the daily routine. On an operational level, privacy is achieved by filtering out unwanted infringements on personal space, but the existential implications of privacy violations are equally important. Like so many other facets of illness, diminished privacy can be experienced as yet another loss and accentuate a sense of diminishing control.

Social Support

Counterbalancing the need for privacy is achieving an optimal level of social support. The need for such support varies from person to person and is usually synchronous with life-long patterns of social connectedness. The importance of social support is so profound that palliative care as a discipline—according to such august bodies as the World Health Organization and the International Association of Hospice and Palliative Care—identifies the patient and family (defined broadly as those who care) as the unit of care. In other words, a dying patient, along with his or her most important social connections, are seen as indivisible from one another within a holistic model of palliative care. As with privacy boundaries, social support can be understood both in terms of its operational importance and its psychological and existential implications. Operationally, the utility of social support is virtually limitless. Extra hands make lighter work, and the work of negotiating life's final months, weeks, or days is often considerable. Social support can supplement many areas of life that illness has placed into deficit. Meals, child care, transportation needs, and housekeeping—the list is as long as the scope of activities and responsibilities that each individual assumes in a state of good health.

The psychological dimensions of social support are equally important but, perhaps, more subtle. Patients with life-threatening and life-limiting illness often experience a fear of abandonment: Will I become too much of a burden? Will my needs become too overwhelming? Will my disease become too disgusting or frightening?

Will I be reduced to a horrible incarnation of my previous self? Any one of these questions may reflect an assumption or fear of abandonment. Besides its operational import, social support provides the much needed assurance: I will not abandon you. Closely aligned with the psychological implications of social support are the existential implications of continuous contact. The meta-message of any form of contact is: You are worthy of my attention and support. Presence, in and of itself, conveys an affirming message of continued care, commitment, investment, and love. Anyone who has ever bemoaned about the "right thing to say" to a critically ill person, need fret no longer. The existential element of social support is fulfilled by simply having shown up.

Care Tenor

Simply put, *care tenor* refers to the tone of care that health care providers offer patients or the tone that patients perceive. For health care providers who wish to deliver dignity-conserving care, the importance of care tenor cannot be overstated. Care tenor denotes everything we convey to patients, besides just our words. Ideally, care tenor should convey the oft-too-little-spoken message and the overarching meta-message of dignity-conserving care: *You matter.* Because each patient matters, he or she deserves care that is accompanied by honor, respect, and esteem. Care tenor can be thought of as the textural component of social support, in that it offers affirmation based on presence. These assertions regarding care tenor are based on one of the key empirical findings in our dignity research: how patients feel they are perceived has substantive influence on their overall sense of dignity.[6,8] The implications for health care, particularly palliative care, are profound.

Restated, the reflection that patients see of themselves in the eye of the beholder—that being the health care provider—should be one that affirms their sense of dignity.[19] Accordingly, those of us in health care must think of ourselves, metaphorically, as a mirror. With every clinical contact, patients gaze our way, looking for an affirming reflection in which can they recognize themselves. If all they see is their illness, they may feel that the essence of who they are has vanished. The less they are able to see of themselves, the more patienthood will have eclipsed personhood. When, in turning to their care providers, patients are able to see a reflection that includes personhood, dignity-conserving care will have been achieved.

There are countless ways that care tenor can be conveyed. Sometimes it is a gentle touch on the shoulder, a look in the eye; mere presence can provide a message of affirmation and respect. The identical message can be received in profoundly different ways, depending on the care tenor that accompanies it. There is a difference between standing at a patient's doorway, rather than sitting in a chair at the bedside.

There is a difference between constantly averting the patient's gaze, rather than maintaining eye contact. There is a difference between being distracted by one's pager, colleagues, students, or even other clinical obligations, rather than being fully present and in the moment with one's patient. Achieving a positive care tenor is usually not a matter of *more* time but the *quality* of time spent with a patient.

It had been a quite evening on the palliative care unit. Dr. J., the Clinical Fellow, had nearly completed her ward rounds. Just prior to dinner, she entered the room of Mr. J., a sixty-eight-year-old man with advanced prostate cancer. All seemed to be in good order; although he was feeling quite weak and fatigued, he was otherwise comfortable. During the course of their meeting, Mr. J.'s meal tray was delivered, which consisted of little more that some clear broth soup. Having a few minutes to spare, Dr. J. sat on his bedside and helped spoon feed him dinner. No words apparently passed between them. But a few minutes later, as she was leaving his room, Mr. J. uttered, "I can never find a way of thanking you for what you've just done for me."

Another way health care providers can be sensitive to care tenor is to consider the A, B, C, and D of dignity-conserving care. This approach is one that I wrote about in the *British Medical Journal* in the summer of 2007.[20] In essence, it makes the case that all health care providers should commit to basic core competencies in the area of whole person, humane, or dignity-conserving care. These competencies can be summarized in the mnemonic A for attitude; B for behavior; C for compassion; and D for dialogue.

Attitude lies at the heart of care tenor and dignity-conserving care. According to the Talmud, "we do not see the world as it is. We see the world as we are." Similarly, we do not necessarily see patients as they are; rather, we see them as we are. How and what we think about our patients is mediated by our attitude toward them. In a study of over two hundred patients within a few months of death, eighty-seven percent of patients associated their personal sense of dignity with the notion of being valued and treated with respect.[5] If attitude provides the lens—depending on its quality and contour—dignity determines the clarity of what is seen.

Behavior refers to the conduct, actions, and deeds health care providers display toward their patients. Invariably, these are outward manifestations of underlying attitudes, which ought to convey a sense of respect and feeling of affirmation. A smile, a touch, a kind gesture of any sort, paying full attention in the moment to each patient; asking permission to perform an examination, using curtains or bedding to safeguard privacy—the list is endless and only limited by the bounds of human decency that one person is willing to show toward another.

Compassion refers to a deep awareness, and the wish to relieve, the suffering of another. Compassion speaks to feelings that are evoked by contact with patients and how those feelings shape our approach to care.[21] Like empathy, compassion is *felt*, not simply processed intellectually. Health care providers arrive at compassion through various means. For some, compassion may be part of a natural disposition that intuitively informs their approach to patient care. For others, compassion emerges from life experience and clinical practice. Compassion may develop gradually over time, with the emerging realization that, like patients, each of us is vulnerable and no one is immune from life's uncertainties. Compassion may also be cultivated by exposure to the humanities (philosophy, ethics, history, and religion), social sciences (anthropology, psychology, sociology), and the arts (literature, theater, film, and visual arts). Each of these disciplines can offer insight into the human condition and the pathos and ambiguity that accompany illness.

Dialogue relates to the nature of conversations that occur between health care providers and patients. The practice of medicine requires the exchange of extensive information within a partnership whose tempo is set by gathering, interpreting, and planning according to new and emerging details. Dialogue is a critical element of the patient experience and dignity-conserving care.[6,8] At its most basic, dialogue must acknowledge whole persons—beyond the illness itself—and recognize the emotional impact that accompanies illness. While busy clinicians often worry, or perhaps rationalize, that these kinds of conversations will take up too much time, that need not be the case. Within the framework of dignity-conserving care, dialogue that acknowledges personhood may be initiated by saying little more than, *This must be frightening for you. I can only imagine what you must be going through. It's natural to feel pretty overwhelmed at times like these.* A question that we have coined the Patient Dignity Question (PDQ) and are just beginning to study asks: What should I know about you as a person that will help me take the best care of you that I can? It is difficult to imagine an area of medicine, from cradle to grave, that would not be well served by an answer to this question, as it taps into elements of personhood that often define core self.

Mr. J., an aboriginal man seen on the palliative care unit, was asked the Patient Dignity Question. The conversation that this precipitated, which took no more than about ten minutes, included the following information:

At the age of eight, he was removed from his family and placed in the residential school system. As a consequence, he was denied the opportunity to get to know his family and to learn his native language. Because of this experience, he always had a hard time trusting people. In fact, he moved countless times during his adult life so as not to let anyone "get too close" to him. To this very day, he struggles with being able to trust people. He wants to, but finds it hard. He sometimes worries that he won't be told the whole truth or that people will see him as not being deserving the whole truth. He is frightened of authority figures. "Those kind of people scare me, but I think I'm getting better than I used to be."

The profound disclosures Mr. J. provides are core to understanding him as a person. The implications of his early childhood experiences and how they shape his outlook on life and experience of patienthood are critically important. Without these insights, it would be easy to see how Mr. J.'s needs might not be met or his sensibilities regarding authority figures and information sharing might be easily offended.

Burden to Others

Illness is fundamentally about loss—loss of health, loss of function, loss of the illusion of invincibility. These losses, large or small, are cumulative and can weigh heavily on patients. The closer that losses align with, or lay claim to, aspects of self that are identified with personhood, the weightier they become. To the dying patient, the question "Am I still me?" is not an intellectual meditation, but rather, a stark expression of personal existential struggle. As the losses mount and the weight becomes crushing, some patients might feel that they are no longer the person they used to be. At its extreme, patients can feel like they no longer serve any particular purpose or function and that life is meaningless. Just as they must shoulder their losses, so, too, they fear, will others have to bear the burden of their inabilities, their dependency, and their neediness.

What happens within the existential landscape of the microbiologist's mind that is no longer able to function in the laboratory? What about the airline pilot who, due to cancer treatment and associated sensory changes, can no longer fly? Or the musician who can no longer play his violin because surgery and postsurgical scarring has impaired his dexterity? As a therapist I have encountered each of these scenarios and countless others. Although the patient may often ask, "What should I do?" the underlying and more profound question is, "Who am I?" In the absence of finding an answer, they might conclude that they are a mere shadow of their former self, the living dead, an inanimate object, or that they are just taking up space. This, in essence, is the mindset of patients who feel themselves a burden to others.

Sensing oneself a burden to others is the equivalent of existential extremis. Western society places profound importance on individual autonomy to the extent that, when it is threatened, personhood itself is felt to be in jeopardy. Sensing oneself a burden to others and devaluing one's life are intimately connected. It is little wonder that nearly every study examining "burden to others" has reported a strong association with a loss of will to live, a desire for death, and outright requests for euthanasia or assisted suicide.[22,23] Among terminally ill patients who actually kill themselves, concerns about being a burden to others are almost universal. Feelings of burden to others has also been linked to quality of life in terminal illness, quality of palliation, and sense of dignity at the end of life.[24]

One of the few studies to specifically examine burden to others among dying patients noted its close association with existential, psychological, and, to a lesser extent, physical symptoms often seen toward the end of life.[24] In our own studies, we reported that about one quarter of terminally ill patients experience a marked sense of burden to others. These feelings are most highly correlated with depression, hopelessness, and quality of life. Of particular note, and far from expected, we did not find an association between sense of burden to others and the degree of actual debility or dependency.[25] It would thus appear that feeling a burden to others is largely mediated through the psychological responses people have to their illness. Dependency, in and of itself, need not lead to feeling a burden to others, so long as psychological resilience is maintained. However, depression and despondency impose a filter through which dependency is conflated with loss of value, neediness, and feeling like a burden. Like self-deprecation, patients who feel that—because of advancing disease and mounting debility—their life no longer has intrinsic meaning or purpose, may assume others will see them similarly. Patients with advanced illness may thus perceive their neediness unfolding in a context shaped by an inability to give anything in return. This perception of needing to take, while having little to give back , epitomizes the psychological landscape of burden to others.

Aftermath Concerns

Although aftermath concerns might be conceived of as a subset of "burden to others," the latter refers to burdens consequent to the illness in the *here and now*, and not those that patients fear may be imposed following their death.[6,8] As a psychiatrist working in palliative care, I have heard many times young fathers worry about how their young family will manage without them. Young mothers, many of whom face life-limiting breast cancers, will lament in anticipation of not being present to guide and nurture their children through an unknowable future. Perhaps the centrality of roles such as being a parent or spouse and death's ability to annihilate those roles heightens the intensity of angst. Rarely is someone's death an event affecting only that individual. Connectedness between human beings means that loss is a communal affair, foisting itself upon all those who love, depend on, and care about the soon to be deceased.

For the most part, addressing aftermath concerns consists of enabling patients to look after, as best they can, the anticipated needs of the soon to be bereft. While it may sound macabre, taking care of one's affairs, writing a will, even making funeral arrangements, can be experienced as ways of attempting to look after loved ones. Although the experience of illness may strip away various roles and the energy or capacity to carry out those roles, it rarely obliterates the ability to care about the people and things that have made life meaningful.

Aftermath concerns can also be addressed in a variety of other ways—providing advice or guidance or offering instruction. Many patient nearing death have written a letter or series of letters in the service of trying to protect and safeguard the well-being of those they will soon leave behind. Perhaps some of the more heart-wrenching and memorable examples of this hearken back to single parents who desperately try to arrange care for their soon to be orphaned children. Their sense of responsibility extends beyond the grave and the solutions they seek must, by definition, somehow transcend the event of their own death. In the coming chapters, we will see how Dignity Therapy may be undertaken in the service of addressing aftermath concerns.

REFERENCES

1. Van Der Maas PJ, Van Delden JJ, Pijnenborg L, Looman CW. Euthanasia and other medical decisions concerning the end of life. *Lancet*. 1991;338(8768):669–674.
2. van der Heide A, Onwuteaka-Philipsen BD, Rurup ML, et al. End-of-life practices in the Netherlands under the Euthanasia Act. *N Engl J Med*. 2007;356(19):1957–1965.
3. Chochinov HM, Wilson KG, Enns M, et al. Desire for death in the terminally ill. *Am J Psychiatry*. 1995;152(8):1185–1191.
4. Chochinov HM, Hack T, Hassard T, Kristjanson LJ, McClement S, Harlos M. Dignity in the terminally ill: a cross-sectional, cohort study. *Lancet*. 2002;360(9350):2026–2030.
5. Chochinov HM, Krisjanson LJ, Hack TF, Hassard T, McClement S, Harlos M. Dignity in the terminally ill: revisited. *J Palliat Med*. 2006;9(3):666–672.
6. Chochinov HM, Hack T, McClement S, Kristjanson L, Harlos M. Dignity in the terminally ill: a developing empirical model. *Soc Sci Med*. 2002;54(3):433–443.
7. Wadensten B, Ahlstrom G. The struggle for dignity by people with severe functional disabilities. *Nurs Ethics*. 2009;16(4):453–465.
8. Chochinov HM. Dignity-conserving care—a new model for palliative care: helping the patient feel valued. *JAMA*. 2002;287(17):2253–2260.
9. Grumann MM, Spiegel D. Living in the face of death: interviews with 12 terminally ill women on home hospice care. *Palliat Support Care*. 2003;1(1):23–32.
10. Sherman DW, Norman R, McSherry CB. A comparison of death anxiety and quality of life of patients with advanced cancer or AIDS and their family caregivers. *J Assoc Nurses AIDS Care*. 2010;21(2):99–112.
11. Erikson EH, ed. *Childhood and society*. New York: Norton; 1950.
12. Buckley J, Herth K. Fostering hope in terminally ill patients. *Nurs Stand*. 2004;19(10): 33–41.
13. Eliott JA, Olver IN. Hope, life, and death: a qualitative analysis of dying cancer patients' talk about hope. *Death Stud*. 2009;33(7):609–638.

14. Chochinov HM, Wilson KG, Enns M, Lander S. Depression, Hopelessness, and suicidal ideation in the terminally ill. *Psychosomatics*. 1998;39(4):366–370.

15. Bauby JD. *The diving bell and the butterfly: a memoir of life in death*. London: Fourth Estate; 1997.

16. Chochinov HM, Hassard T, McClement S, et al. The landscape of distress in the terminally ill. *J Pain Symptom Manage*. 2009;38(5):641–649.

17. Chochinov HM, Tataryn DJ, Wilson KG, Ennis M, Lander S. Prognostic awareness and the terminally ill. *Psychosomatics*. 2000;41(6):500–504.

18. Merriam-Webster Dictionary. *Merriam-Webster Online Dictionary*. Springfield, MA: Merriam-Webster Online; 2005. www.Merriam-Webster.com. Accessed 18 May 2007.

19. Chochinov HM. Dignity and the eye of the beholder. *J Clin Oncol*. 2004;22(7):1336–1340.

20. Chochinov HM. Dignity and the Essence of Medicine: The A, B, C & D of Dignity-Conserving Care. *BMJ*. 2007;335:184–187.

21. Schantz ML. Compassion: a concept analysis. *Nurs Forum*. 2007;42(2):48–55.

22. Ganzini L, Beer TM, Brouns M, Mori M, Hsieh Y.-C. Interest in physician-assisted suicide among Oregon cancer patients, *Journal of Clinical Ethics*. 2006;17:27–28.

23. Sullivan AD, Hedberg K, Fleming DW. Legalized physician-assisted suicide in Oregon—the second year, *New England Journal of Medicine* 2000;342:598–604.

24. Wilson KG, Scott JF, Graham ID, et al. Attitudes of terminally ill patients toward euthanasia and physician-assisted suicide. *Arch Intern Med*. 2000;160(16):2454–2460.

25. Chochinov HM, Kristjanson LJ, Hack TF, Hassard T, McClement S, Harlos M. Burden to others and the terminally ill. *J Pain Symptom Manage*. 2007;34(5):463–471.

2

MOVING DIGNITY INTO CARE

It is more important to know what sort of person has a disease than to know what sort of disease a person has.

—Hippocrates

A successful research program requires being able to follow leads and pursue them in whatever direction the data point. The Model of Dignity in the Terminally Ill, or Dignity Model, described in the previous chapter,[1] represents the first time that researchers have tried to thoroughly study the concept of dignity from the vantage point of dying patients themselves. Although the concept may lack definitional specificity, this does not diminish its importance as a guiding principle of compassionate care. Following the leads embedded in the Dignity Model can help inform best practices in caring for the dying.

The Model of Dignity in the Terminally Ill represents the current understanding of what might influence a dying patient's sense of dignity. Every theme and subtheme in the Dignity Model has a clinical correlate, suggesting an area of attention that might help mitigate suffering for patients nearing death. Together, these clinical correlates constitute what I have called *dignity-conserving care.*[1,2] As previously outlined, the Dignity Model can be divided into three primary areas that address physical (Illness-Related Concerns), existential/spiritual (Dignity-Conserving Repertoire) and social (Social Dignity Inventory) considerations, each bearing on a patient's sense of dignity. The Model of Dignity in the Terminally Ill is not hierarchical; any one or more of its elements may apply within individual circumstances. Although this book focuses on Dignity Therapy, especially as a clinical intervention to address generativity and aftermath concerns, clinicians should be mindful that all the other themes and subthemes in the Dignity Model can inform clinical decisions and define dignity-conserving pathways (see Table 2-1.).[2-4]

The Model of Dignity in the Terminally Ill provides guidance on how to pursue therapeutic approaches by targeting dignity as a viable and achievable outcome. Following the clues embedded in the Dignity Model led to the creation of a novel, individual psychotherapy, now coined *Dignity Therapy*.[2] Various elements of the Dignity Model provide the rationale for each facet of Dignity Therapy, most easily described in terms of *form*, *tone*, and *content*.

HOW THE DIGNITY MODEL INFORMS DIGNITY THERAPY

Form

An important subtheme found in the Dignity Model that shapes the overall form of Dignity Therapy is generativity/legacy. As a developmental task, generativity focuses on investing in those who will outlive us.[5] Attending to generativity means finding ways of prolonging one's influence across time in the service of others. For people who are terminally ill, this means extending aspects of self up to and beyond death itself. As esoteric as this may seem, generativity can be achieved in various simple, concrete ways. Writing a will, planning a funeral, making an advanced directive, or naming a health care proxy are all ways of asserting influence and making one's voice heard, even when it has already been silenced. Each of these generativity strategies can protect survivors from having to make uninformed decisions and thereby safeguard their future well-being. Legacy coupled with generativity can be made tangible, prolonging the influence and sustaining the memory of the deceased in the service of those who survive.

Practitioners of palliative care have begun to recognize the importance of generativity, and how enabling expressions of legacy can mitigate suffering for some patients and certainly for their families. In pediatric palliative care, for instance, clinicians will often arrange to make a handprint of a dying infant or invite the family to save a lock of the child's hair as ways of preserving memories and creating tangible remnants of an all too fleeting life.

The subtheme generativity/legacy arose within the dignity-conserving perspectives domain of the Dignity Model.[1,2] For some patients, feeling that life hasn't stood for anything or that nothing meaningful will be left behind threatens their sense of dignity. Hence, an intervention designed with generativity/legacy in mind facilitates the creation of something that will transcend the patient's death—that is, something that will reflect who they were and what they felt, and express both, when they are no longer here to do so.

Table 2.1 A Model of Dignity and Dignity-Conserving Interventions for Patients Nearing Death

Factors/Subthemes	Dignity-Related Questions	Therapeutic Interventions
Illness-Related Concerns		
Symptom distress		
Physical distress	"How comfortable are you?" "Is there anything we can do to make you more comfortable?"	Vigilance to symptom management Frequent assessment Application of comfort care
Psychological distress	"How are you coping with what is happening to you?"	Assume a supportive stance Empathetic listening Referral to counseling
Medical uncertainty	"Is there anything further about your illness that you would like to know?" "Are you getting all the information you feel you need?"	Upon request, provide accurate, understandable information and strategies to deal with possible future crises
Death anxiety	"Are there things about the later stages of your illness that you would like to discuss?"	
Level of Independence		
Independence	"Has your illness made you more dependent on others?"	Have patients participate in decision making, regarding both medical and personal issues
Cognitive acuity	"Are you having any difficulty with your thinking?"	Treat delirium When possible, avoid sedating medication(s)
Functional capacity	"How much are you able to do for yourself?"	Use orthotics, physiotherapy, and occupational therapy
Dignity-Conserving Repertoire		
Dignity-conserving perspectives		
Continuity of self	"Are there things about you that this disease does not affect?"	Acknowledge and take interest in those aspects of the patient's life that he or she most values See the patient as worthy of honor, respect, and esteem

Table 2.1 (Continued)

Factors/Subthemes	Dignity-Related Questions	Therapeutic Interventions
Role preservation	"What things did you do before you were sick that were most important to you?"	
Maintenance of pride	"What about yourself or your life are you most proud of?"	
Hopefulness	"What is still possible?"	Encourage and enable the patient to participate in meaningful or purposeful activities
Autonomy/control	"How in control do you feel?"	Involve patient in treatment and care decisions
Generativity/legacy	"How do you want to be remembered?"	Life project (e.g., making audio/video tapes, writing letters, journaling) Dignity Psychotherapy
Acceptance	"How at peace are you with what is happening to you?"	Support the patient in his or her outlook Encourage doing things that enhance his or her sense of well-being (e.g., meditation, light exercise, listening to music, prayer)
Resilience/fighting spirit	"What part of you is strongest right now?"	
Dignity-conserving practices		
Living in the moment	"Are there things that take your mind away from illness and offer you comfort?"	Allow the patient to participate in normal routines or take comfort in momentary distractions (e.g., daily outings, light exercise, listening to music)
Maintaining normalcy	"Are there things you still enjoy doing on a regular basis?"	
Finding spiritual comfort	"Is there a religious or spiritual community that you are, or would like to be, connected with?"	Make referrals to chaplain or spiritual leader Enable the patient to participate in particular spiritual and/or culturally based practices

(continued)

Table 2.1 (Continued)

Factors/Subthemes	Dignity-Related Questions	Therapeutic Interventions
Social Dignity Inventory		
Privacy boundaries	"What about your privacy or your body is important to you?"	Ask permission to examine patient Proper draping to safeguard and respect privacy
Social support	"Who are the people that are most important to you?" "Who is your closest confidante?"	Liberal policies about visitation, rooming in Enlist involvement of a wide support network
Care tenor	"Is there anything in the way you are treated that is undermining your sense of dignity?"	Treat the patient as worthy of honor, esteem, and respect; adopt a stance conveying this
Burden to others	"Do you worry about being a burden to others?" "If so, to whom and in what ways?"	Encourage explicit discussion about these concerns with those they fear they are burdening
Aftermath concerns	"What are your biggest concerns for the people you will leave behind?"	Encourage the settling of affairs, preparation of an advanced directive, making a will, funeral planning

For reasons that will be elaborated in later chapters, the written word is an ideal mode of generativity/legacy. Therefore, Dignity Therapy[1,3,6] involves the creation of a document—a carefully constructed and edited document—consisting of content that patients would want known by those they are about to leave behind. This document, or *Generativity Document,* is a vital component of Dignity Therapy. Its significance is two-fold: first, it conveys a sense of profound regard for the disclosures patients share, in the moment, during their Dignity Therapy; and second, it ensures that whatever is said is captured and preserved for posterity.

Tone

The term *dignity* means "to be worthy of honor, respect, and esteem."[7] As such, Dignity Therapy must convey respect and a tone of sincere affirmation for each of its participants. While *generativity* has an ethereal quality pertaining to sometime in the future, the *tone* of Dignity Therapy needs to be experienced in the here and now. Care tenor, subsumed within the Social Dignity Inventory, is the Dignity Model subtheme that most clearly informs the tone of Dignity Therapy.[2]

Our studies have shown that care tenor, or the *tone of care,* has a profound influence on patient sense of dignity. One of our earliest studies, published in *The Lancet,*[8] reported that appearance, or *how patients experience themselves to be seen* by their health care providers, is the most ardent predictor of sense of dignity. It is reasonable to infer that these perceptions, in large measure, are based on care tenor. Dignity affirming care tenor refers to the multitude of ways that health care providers convey appreciation, respect, and kindness to their patients. It may be a gentle touch, taking the time to sit at the bedside, or even the subtleties of body language that convey the message: *You are a whole person and deserve my time, my respect, and my care.* Practitioners of Dignity Therapy must always be mindful of their care tenor and its influence on patients. Even a beautifully edited, accurate, and complete generativity document cannot salvage an experience of Dignity Therapy wherein patients' preferences, stories, experiences, and disclosures have not been treated with respect.

The care tenor that should typify Dignity Therapy is closely approximated by Carl Rogers' Client-Centered Therapy (CCT).[9] Rogers described three critical attitudes for CCT therapists, including genuineness, unconditional positive regard, and empathic understanding. Genuineness refers to therapists being able to show themselves as real, authentic persons, not hiding behind a professional façade of impersonality. Unconditional positive regard means that the therapist shows complete acceptance of the patient, displaying consistent and nonjudgmental care. Therapists demonstrate empathic understanding when they try to connect with and appreciate their patients, by way of attentive listening and sensitivity to what patients are trying to say. Each of these attitudes will serve the Dignity Therapist well: therapists need to show genuine and personal interest in patients and what they have to say; therapists need to show unconditional positive regard for patients and be nonjudgment in eliciting the story patients need to share; and therapists need to be empathic as a way of connecting with, and providing affirmation for, their patients.

Tone is easier to observe or feel than to describe. However, its importance cannot be overstated. While therapists try to discern what patients are thinking or feeling, patients attempt to read the subtle clues exhibited by their therapist; *Am I an engaging patient? "Are you interested in what I have to say? Am I doing this right? How does my story compare to others you've heard?* If patients feel that they are somehow failing or disappointing the therapist, the experience of personal disclosure will begin to feel assaultive, perhaps even demeaning, quickly leading to disenchantment and therapeutic disengagement. Therapists must be genuine and enthusiastic partners within the collaborative effort it takes to accomplish successful Dignity Therapy. Hence, therapists must always remember: everyone has an important and unique story to tell, feigned interest is readily transparent, and nothing is more encouraging to a storyteller than an engaged listener.

Content

Here again, the Dignity Model provides vital clues on shaping the content of Dignity Therapy.[1,2] Dignity Therapy is facilitated by a series of questions (see chapter 3). The themes informing these questions derive from dignity-conserving perspectives and aftermath concerns. Dignity-conserving perspectives contain the subthemes continuity of self, role preservation, maintenance of pride, hopefulness (understood, on the basis of qualitative analysis, to denote a sense of meaning or purpose) and autonomy/control. Each of these subthemes represents an aspect of psychological and existential makeup or outlook, having a bearing on the patient's sense of dignity and resonating with a sense of core self. Thus, the Dignity Therapy question framework is designed to elicit information that highlights the importance of these areas and invites patients to address those they deem to be most salient or meaningful.[2,3,10]

Aftermath concerns also inform the content of Dignity Therapy, allowing patients to address issues that they anticipate will arise in the wake of their death. Perhaps there are specific instructions they might want to leave, or words of wisdom or guidance they might like to share with particular individuals. Being mindful of aftermath concerns means providing patients appropriate openings to broach these delicate, often poignant, areas of inquiry.[2,3,10,11]

DIGNITY THERAPY REVEALED

The confluence of form, tone, and content led to the creation of a novel individualized psychotherapy, especially intended for patients nearing the end of life. We coined this psychotherapy, *Dignity Therapy*, given that each element of this therapeutic approach is based on the Model of Dignity in the Terminally Ill.[1,2] In essence, patients taking part in Dignity Therapy are invited to engage in conversations, addressing issues or memories that they deem important or that they want recorded for the sake of those loved ones who will outlive them.[2,3] In the service of generativity, the conversations are audio-recorded and transcribed. Hence, the therapy results in the creation of something that will last—something whose influence will extend beyond the death of the patient, to be heard across coming generations. The role of the therapist, besides guiding and enabling the process, is to imbue the therapeutic interaction with dignity; this means that patients must feel accepted, valued, and honored.

The first inkling that Dignity Therapy might be a viable and, indeed, a special palliative care intervention emerged with the very first study participant. The details of his story will be told elsewhere,[12] but the fact that he decided life was still worth living "at least until this [Dignity Therapy] can be done" was an auspicious beginning for the Dignity Therapy clinical trials. Early promise led to rapid success in securing research funding with support coming from the American Foundation for Suicide Prevention, the National Cancer Institute of Canada, and the Canadian Institutes of Health Research.

During the course of the first clinical trial that ran between 2001 and 2003, the idea of Dignity Therapy entered the literature with an article entitled "Dignity Conserving Care—A New Model for Palliative Care." This article, published May 1, 2002 in the *Journal of the American Medical Association*,[2] provides a detailed explanation of the Model of Dignity in the Terminally Ill and introduces readers to Mr. S., a Dignity Therapy participant. Mr. S. was a sixty-two-year-old man with primary lung cancer who, eighteen months earlier, had been diagnosed with metastases to his liver, brain, and adrenal glands. He had recently developed severe weakness of the left upper and lower extremities, with an inability to bear weight. He had discontinued steroids because of unpleasant side effects and completed a two-week course of antibiotics for pneumonia. His symptoms, including shortness of breath, seizures, constipation, and occasional agitation, were relatively well controlled. Lately, the focus of his management had become comfort care.

Mr. S. used the occasion of his Dignity Therapy to recount various early-life struggles encountered within his adoptive family.[2] Sadly, he never felt a sense of belonging, which led to chronic self-loathing behavior, chaotic relationships, innumerable vocational mishaps, and a string of addictions. This self-destructive pathway was miraculously interrupted when he met the woman who later became his wife. As a result of their love and the healing it promoted, he was rescued from drug abuse, alcoholism, and, ultimately, from himself. For Mr. S., Dignity Therapy provided both the chance to thank his wife for "saving" him and an opportunity to leave behind a tale of hope for anyone following a similar, destructive course. Upon receiving his generativity document, Mrs. S remarked, "Being able to read his words will be a way of helping me to remember him, and to think of him. I didn't always understand him, because he was a free spirit and I was the worrier. Maybe I didn't trust God enough. I'm glad I'll have his words to comfort me."

THE FIRST CLINICAL TRIAL IS PUBLISHED

In August 2005, the results of the first clinical trial of Dignity Therapy were published in the *Journal of Clinical Oncology*.[10] An accompanying editorial by Betty

Ferrell hailed it as a "major breakthrough" for palliative care.[13] In the study, Dignity Therapy was offered to all patients registered to receive palliative care services in Perth, Australia and Winnipeg, Canada, meeting a priori eligibility criteria. In Australia, patients were recruited from the Silver Chain Hospice Care Service and the Cancer Council Centre for Palliative Care Cottage Hospice. In Canada, patients were recruited from the Winnipeg Regional Health Authority Palliative Care Program. In both Winnipeg and Perth, the palliative care programs offer a broad range of inpatient and outpatient services.

To be eligible for the study, patients had to have a terminal illness with a life expectancy of no more than six months, be a minimum of eighteen years of age, speak English, be willing to commit to three to four contacts over approximately seven to ten days, be cognitively intact, and be willing to provide verbal and written consent. To evaluate the efficacy of Dignity Therapy, all participants were asked to fill out questionnaires measuring a wide range of physical, psychological, and existential issues and concerns, including depression, dignity, anxiety, suffering, hopelessness, desire for death, suicide, sense of well-being, quality of life, and will to live. Once the questionnaires were completed, patients took part in Dignity Therapy.[10] They were asked to speak on audiotape about what mattered most to them, including what they would want to say to the people closest to them. (The specific protocol and techniques used to facilitate these discussions are described in later chapters.)

Over a two-year period, 100 patients completed the study, evenly spit between Australia and Canada. Most of these patients had advanced, end-stage cancer, with a median survival of fifty-one days from the first point of contact to the time of death. Of the 100 patients who completed the study, 91% reported feeling satisfied or highly satisfied with the Dignity Therapy; 86% reported that the intervention was helpful or very helpful. Seventy-six percent indicated that it heightened their sense of dignity; 68% indicated that Dignity Therapy increased their sense of purpose; and 67% indicated that it heightened their sense of meaning. Forty-seven percent of participants indicated that dignity therapy increased their will to live. One sixty-two-year-old woman with metastatic breast cancer went so far as to say, "I see [taking part in this study] as one reason why I am alive." Eighty-one percent of patients completing Dignity Therapy reported that it had already helped, or would help, their family.[10]

Participants used Dignity Therapy in a variety of ways. For some, it offered the ability to affirm their love for friends and family members, while for others, there were expressions of regret. For most patients, Dignity Therapy was an opportunity to recount memories of special life events and moments of celebration or of tragedy; often, these were moments that had changed, defined, or shaped their lives. Many patients raised issues related to the theme of generativity; for example, one thirty-six-year-old woman dying of metastatic breast cancer said, "I'm very happy to have participated in this project. It's helped bring my memories, thoughts, and feelings into perspective instead of all jumbled emotions running through my head. The most important thing has been that I'm able to leave a sort of 'insight' of myself for my husband and children and all my family and friends." For other patients, Dignity Therapy offered a chance to reaffirm their sense of continued self-worth. One forty-nine-year-old woman with end-stage breast cancer stated, "Dignity Therapy was a lovely experience. Getting down on paper what I thought was a dull, boring life really opened my eyes to how much I really have done."[10]

Another patient, a sixty-one-year-old woman with a recurrent rectal cancer, captured the essence of hopefulness as it relates to issues of ongoing meaning and purpose: "This experience has helped me to delve within myself and see more meaning to my life. I really look forward to sharing it with my family. I have no doubt that it will be enlightening to them." The wife of a seventy-two-year-old man with end-stage lung cancer described the transcript as "magnificent," indicating that her husband "wanted to contribute; the interview gave him a 'second chance' to do something to help."[10] Given how prominent and existentially crippling "feeling a burden to others" can be for patients,[8,14] providing an opportunity to invoke meaning and purpose—to help patients feel that life might amount to more than mere existence—can be a salve to the spirit. Health care professionals should take note of these opportunities and use every clinical encounter as a chance to acknowledge, reinforce, and, where possible, affirm the personhood of patients charged to their care.[15]

In this study,[10] measures of suffering and depression also showed significant improvements. Measures of dignity, hopelessness, desire for death, anxiety, will to live, and suicide all showed changes favoring improvement. Patients who initially reported more despair were also more likely to benefit from Dignity Therapy. Patients who found Dignity Therapy to be helpful were significantly more likely to report that their lives felt meaningful, that they had a heightened sense of purpose and will to live, and that they experienced less suffering. Those who believed that Dignity Therapy had, or would, help their families, were significantly more likely to experience life as meaningful and purposeful, and to report greater will to live and less suffering. This is one of those thought-provoking findings when an insight, coming from an end-of-life perspective, reflects an essential truth resonating across the human life cycle. People who are able to safeguard, in some measure, the well-being of something or someone they care about, are more likely to embrace life and its sense of meaning and purpose. This is true throughout life and, according to the data, appears to be sustained until its very end.[10]

The rationale for many palliative care interventions is to make a patient less aware of his or her suffering. Although analgesia does not eliminate the source of physical pain, it nevertheless effectively eliminates the sensation of pain. Dignity Therapy, however, attempts to deal with emotional pain by targeting its source. It attempts to bolster a sense of meaning and purpose, while reinforcing a continued sense of worth within a framework that is supportive, nurturing, and accessible, even for those proximate to death. The benefits of Dignity Therapy and its viability as an end-of-life intervention were wholly supported by the results of this first study.[10]

WHAT ABOUT FAMILIES?

Like patients, families are deeply affected by the experience of anticipatory loss and impending death. Patient and family suffering frequently overlap, with loved ones often vicariously experiencing the patient's distress. The field of palliative care now includes families and patients as the unit of care. Hence, palliative care practitioners strive to improve quality of life, both for people nearing death and those who will soon grieve them. Although the lived experience of patients and families is very different, there are some interesting areas of overlap. Loss is a common denominator; so, too, are some of the critical dynamics pertaining to dignity. For patients, loss of dignity, sense of personhood, and notions of affirmation are finely interwoven. Like patients, families suffer when they feel that their loved ones have been reduced to "what they have" rather than "who they are." Hence, the very dynamic that undermines patients' sense of dignity is apt to cause distress for family members. That being the case, factors that affirm patient dignity often have a similar effect on families.

To explore the influence of Dignity Therapy on families, we spoke with recipients of Dignity Therapy generativity documents nine to twelve months after the death of their loved ones.[16] This time frame was chosen to allow resolution of the acute phases of grief, while still providing adequate proximity to the loss to enable accurate recall. Of the 100 patients who completed the previously described Phase I Dignity Therapy trial, sixty family members provided feedback on their experience of this intervention. This group primarily consisted of spouses and adult children. As was the case with patients, the family data from this study overwhelmingly affirmed the benefits of this novel therapeutic approach. Ninety-five percent of family members felt that Dignity Therapy had helped their loved one, with one daughter observing, "Mom was extremely closed emotionally and had huge difficulties expressing her feelings. This gave her an opportunity to do so without feeling vulnerable." Seventy-eight percent of family members reported that Dignity Therapy had heightened their loved one's sense of dignity, and 72% reported that it had enhanced the patient's sense of purpose. A daughter described her father's experience in this way: "He had something to say, wanted to be heard, wanted to pass on a message of hope. It helped him find some value in what he had done and remember who he was." Sixty-five percent of family members felt that Dignity Therapy had helped their loved one prepare for death; that same proportion also indicated that Dignity Therapy had been as important a component of palliative care as anything other aspect of the patient's care. For a short, individualized, nonpharmacological intervention, this finding is particularly striking.

The benefits of Dignity Therapy were expressed by family members in a variety of ways.[16] Some felt that Dignity Therapy affirmed their loved one's sense of purpose and feelings of having lived a worthwhile life. One daughter observed, "Reading the document gave my Mom a sense of accomplishment. I believe, It gave her a tangible way of looking back at a life well lived." Many families reported that the idea of leaving something behind had particular resonance for their departed loved one. One woman said this of her late husband: "He felt that our grandsons, including our latest whom unfortunately he never lived to see, would get some idea of his life and what he had achieved." In a similar vein, a family member underscored how "[Dignity Therapy] legitimizes your life and provides an opportunity to put down on paper what you hope is your legacy."[16]

Family members also felt Dignity Therapy influenced their grief and accommodation to loss. Seventy-eight percent of family members reported that the generativity document helped them in their time of grief and that the document remained a source of comfort for them and other members of their family. A daughter had this to say: "I would say it was more helpful than any mourning aspect. It helped me move past it. Family and friends are certainly a support but through the document, my Mom was also able to provide support." Another daughter described it as "something to hold onto at the time of Dad's passing and it made Dad's life and ways alive and tender." Summarizing the benefits for both patients and families, one family member had this to say: "I think the Dignity Therapy truly helped him feel as though he were doing something useful and to be able to leave behind a part of himself. That in turn has helped myself and the children as it is almost like receiving a special gift of his words that we can have for our life time." [16]

Although most feedback from families was positive, it is important to point out that three recipients of generativity documents felt dissatisfied. In one instance, a wife was concerned that some material contained in the document might be hurtful to her husband's siblings.[16] The protocol is extremely rigorous in protecting against this kind of occurrence, but in this instance, someone who did not have permission to access it had taken the document. The other examples of dissatisfaction pertain to feelings that the document did not accurately capture who the person had really been. In order to avoid creating a distortion of the participant—something that practitioners of Dignity Therapy must always be mindful of—exclusionary criteria such as confusion, marked depression, or simply being too ill to provide thoughtful and meaningful responses must thoroughly be evaluated and applied. Interestingly, some family members were present during Dignity Therapy; however, none of the dissatisfied family members were present or participated in the process of Dignity Therapy.[16] In our experience, the presence of a family member can provide quality assurance, ensuring that responses are consistent with who the patient is; family members can also offer suggestions that can cue or facilitate meaningful and fulsome disclosures.

GOLD STANDARD EVIDENCE

The status quo is difficult to change. This is a truism in many areas of life, particularly in medicine. Commonly held practices are hard to displace, with change only happening in the face of new and convincing evidence. When it comes to humane care and how patients are treated, challenging the status quo can be very difficult. Medicine has become so technologically and biologically focused that the way we behave toward patients is seen as incidental—the niceties of care, so to speak, having little if anything to do with care itself. Typically, clinicians' behavior is intuitive, based on individual personality characteristics and, in some instances, shaped by the approach of previous mentors. Sometimes this works, and other times, it doesn't.

Our own research on dignity has shown, *empirically*, that the way care providers, including physicians, behave toward patients—their ability to affirm patients as whole persons—is a powerful mediator of patient and family satisfaction.[8,12] This certainly validates Francis Peabody's famous aphorism, "The secret of the care of the patient is in caring for the patient."[17] Yet it is no secret that psychosocial aspects of care are often given short shrift and even considered beyond the purview of medicine. As convincing as the first study of Dignity Therapy was, its ability to influence patient care and change practice among ardent empiricists may be limited. After all, a phase I study does not test an intervention against a control group. It could be argued that the mere presence of an empathic person may have been the only salutary element of Dignity Therapy. While the robustness and poignancy of the data suggests otherwise, for some, nothing short of a randomized controlled trial merits attention or sways practice.

On the basis of the strong phase I Dignity Therapy data, our research group received funds from the National Institutes of Health, based in Bethesda, Maryland. Between 2004 and 2008, with colleagues from Perth, Australia, led by Dr. Linda Kristjanson, and from New York City, led by Dr. William Breitbart, we conducted a three-country, three-arm randomized controlled trial. Participants were eligible if they had a life expectancy of six months or less and were registered with the palliative care program affiliated with their particular recruitment site. Participants also needed to be eighteen years of age or older, able to commit to three to four contacts over about seven to ten days, and willing to provide written informed consent. As in our phase I trial, participants were excluded if they were cognitively impaired, too unwell to complete the requirements of the protocol, or unable to speak English.

Once the study had been explained and consent was obtained, participants were randomly assigned to one of three study arms:

- Dignity Therapy, as previously described.
- Client-Centered Care (CCC): Participants randomized to Client-Centered Care were invited to take part in a conversation focused on here-and-now issues. To keep the conversations within specified parameters, participants were asked about their illness, associated symptoms, and actions taken to make them more comfortable. Unlike Dignity Therapy, CCC did not explore themes related to meaning and purpose, nor did it result in the creation of a generativity document. The primary aim of this study arm was to replicate the frequency and amount of contact that patients had with an empathic interviewer, thereby controlling for the effect of increased attention.
- Standard care: Participants assigned to standard care had access to the full range of palliative care support services available to all non-study patients. Those assigned to standard care completed baseline psychological measures and then, seven to ten days later—the time frame that approximated the first and last contact of participants in the other two study arms—all additional study measures were administered and completed.

This study used a broad range of standard measures, including the Spiritual Wellbeing Scale (FACIT-Sp);[18] Patient Dignity Inventory;[19] Hospital Anxiety and Depression Scale;[20] and several items from the Structured Interview for Symptoms and Concerns,[21] including dignity, desire for death, suffering, hopelessness, depression, suicidal ideation, and sense of burden to others. A standard measure of physical symptom distress (The Edmonton Symptom Assessment Scale)[22] was also administered. Because of concerns about low initial levels of distress, a poststudy survey, identical across all three arms, was administered to every study participant.

In August 2011, our research group published its findings in *Lancet Oncology*. Three hundred twenty six patients with a terminal prognosis were randomized across the three study conditions. Because of initial low base rates of distress, no significant differences were noted in pre versus post study measures in any of the groups. However, the post study survey revealed marked differences between the three study arms. Patients reported that dignity therapy was significantly more likely than the other two interventions to have been helpful, improve quality of life, increase sense of dignity, change how their family saw and appreciated them, and be helpful to their family. Dignity therapy was significantly better than client-centred care in improving spiritual wellbeing, and was significantly better than standard palliative care in terms of lessening sadness or depression; significantly more patients who had received dignity therapy reported that the study group had been satisfactory, compared with those who received standard palliative care.

To date, hundreds if not thousands of patients—and their family members—have taken part in Dignity Therapy in Canada, the United States, Australia, China, Japan, England, Scotland, Denmark, Portugal and Sweden, to name but a few places where clinical trials of Dignity Therapy are taking place. Several studies have recently been published, reporting on the performance of Dignity Therapy under various circumstances. A Danish study of ten health care professionals and twenty patients concluded that, with minor cultural adaptations, Dignity Therapy was a manageable, acceptable, and relevant intervention for Danish patients admitted to palliative care.[23] Another study of eight patients with end stage cancer showed that Dignity Therapy could be delivered by telemedicine and achieve overall benefit and high levels of patient satisfaction.[24] A recently published study conducted in French Canada reported that within a cohort of thirty-three dying patients, relevance and satisfaction were found to be high for patients and families alike.[25]

While the quantitative data continues to mount, the value of Dignity Therapy is perhaps best revealed by the stories of those who have experienced it. In many instances, the stories share simple wisdom that people wish to pass along to their loved ones. For instance, a sixty-three-year-old woman and mother of three grown children participated in Dignity Therapy three months before dying of colon cancer. She reminisced about the virtues of her own marriage and how she had worked hard to make it better than so many unsuccessful marriages she had seen in her own family: "you have to have the physical, but you also have to combine that with the friendship part." Within her generativity document, she was able to say, how "very proud" she was of each of her children. "I'm very pleased on how they turned out. I was worried when they were teenagers, but they turned out to be great people." She was able to tell her family that she was happy with how her own life had turned out, perhaps making it easier for her to share this parting wisdom: "Just be happy and lead the happiest life that you can. Be peaceful with yourself. Nobody has a perfect life, but still, figure out things in your own life and be the happiest that you can be."

A middle-aged, single teacher with end-stage gastroesophageal cancer was able to share the pride he took in helping shape the lives of his young students. He summarized his approach to teaching as follows: "Be kind. Find how you can help them and be there to help them help themselves; not always to do things for them, but to help themselves. Be honest and fair with people. Then you need never be ashamed."

In choosing his final, parting words for his family—an aging mother and older brother—he said, "Don't despair and look after each other."

In addition to other purposes, many patients have used Dignity Therapy to give their spouse explicit permission to remarry. One fifty-two-year-old woman said, "I don't want to see him on his own for the rest of his life, because he will need a lot of support himself. He will have his family, of course, but he may still need a companion in his life and possibly even build a different life. Yes, I would like him to be happy, to find happiness later." On one occasion, a father used Dignity Therapy to encourage his son to "exercise and lose a few pounds." He went on to say, "I'd like to tell my family how much I love them, and tell my kids that they can achieve whatever they want to achieve in life." During the course of her Dignity Therapy, one elderly woman tried to explain how her conflicted relationship with her sister had led to her emotional disengagement from her nephews. In her final weeks of life, she saw this as an opportunity, if not to fully reconcile—something that she realized might be too late—at the very least to provide them with an explanation.

Time and time again, Dignity Therapy has captured pivotal moments in life—moments such as births, marriages, deaths, even first meetings—when, for that individual, time stood still and memories were indelibly etched. One gentleman, sixty years after the fact, gaily recalled the first time he caught a glimpse of the woman who would later become his wife. An elderly, retired journalist remembered being a few feet away from the dais when the results confirming Pierre Elliot Trudeau's victory as leader of Canada's Federal Liberal Party were announced. Another memory, fixed in the mind of a seventy-six-year-old woman with advanced cancer, was of her father being killed in France during the Allied invasion of Normandy. She recalled how "a soldier came to bring the letter for my mother, but she wasn't home. She was working, and I got it. Of course, I opened the letter and read it. I didn't show it to my mother for a week. I didn't know how to and when I did tell her, she cried and cried. I'll never forget that." By including it as part of her Dignity Therapy, the story, no doubt, will be passed along from one generation to the next.

TIME TO MOVE ON

At this point, readers should understand the basis of Dignity Therapy, the research that provides its foundation, and the basic form of the intervention itself. Moreover, readers should be aware of how empiricism has shaped Dignity Therapy, along with the rigorous data that support its application as a novel, viable, and effective palliative care intervention. There is good evidence that Dignity Therapy can enhance end of life experience for people nearing death; it can improve spiritual well being and, in some instances, quality of life. Dignity Therapy can enhance a dying patient's sense of dignity. Dignity therapy can help patients cope with disappointments, process the reality of leaving behind loved ones, deal with feelings of sadness, loss, isolation, and a damaged sense of identity and personal value. It can also help patients consider personal priorities in terms of relationships, religious and spiritual beliefs, and deal with the urgency of resolving conflicts or achieve personally meaningful goals. And for family members, Dignity Therapy can assuage feelings of grief and provide a comforting presence during their time of loss.

Why is such extensive and detailed background information on Dignity Therapy so important? Because new treatment fads are all too common, causing the public to become wary and medical professionals outright skeptical. Therefore, anyone planning to administer Dignity Therapy must know—and their patients and their patients' care providers must know—that in delivering this form of therapy, they are standing on solid empirical ground. The solidity of that foundation can provide patients, families, and care providers the assurance that their treatment is evidence-based, that the data supporting Dignity Therapy in a palliative care population are strong, and that Dignity Therapy may very well help mitigate various kinds of distress or suffering that patients and families face within the context of palliative care.

REFERENCES

1. Chochinov HM, Hack T, McClement S, Kristjanson L, Harlos M. Dignity in the terminally ill: a developing empirical model. *Soc Sci Med.* 2002;54(3):433–443.
2. Chochinov HM. Dignity-conserving care—a new model for palliative care: helping the patient feel valued. *JAMA.* 2002;287(17):2253–2260.
3. McClement SE, Chochinov HM, Hack TF, Kristjanson LJ, Harlos M. Dignity-conserving care: application of research findings to practice. *Int J Palliat Nurs.* 2004;10(4):173–179.
4. Chochinov HM. Dying, dignity, and new horizons in palliative end-of-life care. *CA Cancer J Clin.* 2006;56(2):84–103.
5. Erikson EH, ed. *Childhood and society.* New York: Norton; 1950.
6. Chochinov HM, Hack T, Hassard T, Kristjanson LJ, McClement S, Harlos M. Dignity and psychotherapeutic considerations in end-of-life care. *J Palliat Care.* 2004;20(3):134–142.
7. Merriam-Webster Dictionary. *Merriam-Webster Online Dictionary.* Springfield, MA: Merriam-Webster Online; 2005. www.Merriam-Webster.com. Accessed 18 May 2007.
8. Chochinov HM, Hack T, Hassard T, Kristjanson LJ, McClement S, Harlos M. Dignity in the terminally ill: a cross-sectional, cohort study. *Lancet.* 2002;360(9350):2026–2030.
9. Rogers CR. *Client-centered therapy; its current practice, implications, and theory.* Oxford, England: Houghton Mifflin; 1951.
10. Chochinov HM, Hack T, Hassard T, Kristjanson LJ, McClement S, Harlos M. Dignity therapy: a novel psychotherapeutic intervention for patients near the end of life. *J Clin Oncol.* 2005;23(24):5520–5525.
11. Wilson KG, Curran D, McPherson CJ. A burden to others: a common source of distress for the terminally ill. *Cogn Behav Ther.* 2005;34(2):115–123.
12. Chochinov HM. Dignity and the eye of the beholder. *J Clin Oncol.* 2004;22(7):1336–1340.

13. Ferrell, B. Dignity Therapy: Advancing the science of spiritual care in terminal illness. *J Clin Oncol.* 2005;23: 5427–5428.
14. Chochinov HM, Kristjanson LJ, Hack TF, Hassard T, McClement S, Harlos M. Burden to others and the terminally ill. *J Pain Symptom Manage.* 2007;34(5):463–471.
15. Chochinov HM. Dignity and the Essence of Medicine: The A, B, C & D of Dignity-Conserving Care. *BMJ.* 2007;335:184–187.
16. McClement S, Chochinov HM, Hack T, Hassard T, Kristjanson LJ, Harlos M. Dignity therapy: family member perspectives. *J Palliat Med.* 2007;10(5):1076–1082.
17. Peabody FW. A medical classic: the care of the patient. *JAMA.* 1927;88:877.
18. Peterman AH, Fitchett G, Brady MJ, Hernandez L, Cella D. Measuring spiritual well-being in people with cancer: the functional assessment of chronic illness therapy—Spiritual Well-being Scale (FACIT-Sp). *Ann Behav Med.* 2002;24(1):49–58.
19. Chochinov HM, Hassard T, McClement SE, et al. The Patient Dignity Inventory: A novel way of measuring dignity-related distress in palliative care. *J Pain Symptom Manage.* 2008;36:559–571.
20. Zigmond AS, Snaith RP. The hospital anxiety and depression scale. *Acta Psychiatr Scand.* 1983;67(6):361–370.
21. Wilson KG, Graham ID, Viola RA, et al. Structured interview assessment of symptoms and concerns in palliative care. *Can J Psychiatry.* 2004;49(6):350–358.
22. Bruera E, Kuehn N, Miller MJ, Selmser P, Macmillan K. The Edmonton Symptom Assessment System (ESAS): a simple method for the assessment of palliative care patients. *J Palliat Care.* 1991;7(2):6–9.
23. Houmann LJ, Rydahl-Hansen S, Chochinov HM, Kristjanson LJ, Groenvold M. Testing the feasibility of the Dignity Therapy interview: adaptation for the Danish culture. BMC Palliat Care. 2010;9:21.
24. Passik SD, Kirsh KL, Leibee S, Kaplan LS, Love C, Napier E, Burton D, Sprang R. A feasibility study of dignity psychotherapy delivered via telemedicine. Palliat Support Care. 2004;2:149–55.
25. Gagnon P, Chochinov HM, Cochrane J, Le Moignan Moreau J, Fontaine R, Croteau L. *Psychothérapie de la Dignité*: Une intervention pour réduire la détresse psychologique chez les personnes en soins palliatifs. Psycho-Oncologie. 2010; 4 :169–175.
26. Harvey Max Chochinov, Linda J Kristjanson, William Breitbart, Susan McClement, Thomas F Hack, Tom Hassard, Mike Harlos Effect of dignity therapy on distress and end-of-life experience in terminally ill patients: a randomised controlled trial. Lancet Oncol. 2011;12:753-62.

3

INTRODUCING DIGNITY THERAPY TO PATIENTS AND FAMILIES

The secret of the care of the patient is in caring for the patient.

—Francis W. Peabody

Until now, we have discussed the theoretical foundations of Dignity Therapy. The importance that clinicians place on this background material will vary. However, anyone intending to practice Dignity Therapy should know that the intervention itself is based on sound research and that the efficacy of this approach has been examined for patients facing life-threatening and life-limiting conditions.[1-5] Most clinicians want to know that the therapeutic approaches they offer patients are evidence-based and not simply based on intuition or good intentions. Being aware of this empirical foundation will comfort practitioners and recipients of Dignity Therapy alike. As important, it will shape how health care professionals view Dignity Therapy as they consider making this novel intervention available to their patients nearing the end of life.

PATIENT SELECTION FOR DIGNITY THERAPY

> **Step 1.** The first step is to determine which patients might benefit from Dignity Therapy. This means understanding eligibility criteria and knowing which patients should not take part.

Like any therapeutic modality, knowing when to apply it and when not to apply it is of utmost importance (see Step 1 box). When Dignity Therapy was first being developed, we assumed that it would be best suited for people expressing significant distress, particularly within the realm of psychosocial or existential discomfort. Recall that Dignity Therapy was developed to promote generativity and provide a tangible, important life task for people nearing death. It thus seemed likely that this approach would apply especially well to individuals whose distress was marked by a paucity of meaning and purpose in the final months, weeks, and days of life.

While it is hard to miss physical distress, experience has taught us that suffering and existential torment can sometimes be less obvious to the observer. This does not make them any less important causes of distress within the palliative care setting. For instance, Mr. J was a fifty-four-year-old successful businessman, recently diagnosed with an inoperable pancreatic tumor. Although his physical symptoms had been well controlled on the palliative care unit, his attending physician was surprised to hear him describe his suffering as "intolerable." When asked to explain, he expressed a sense of deep despair, which came from knowing that his time was limited, that he was being forced to relinquish the control he had always maintained in his professional and personal life, and that he would soon leave his wife and young family behind.

If this gentleman had not specifically been asked about the sources of his anguish, his suffering may very well have gone unnoticed. This underscores the importance of *always testing our assumptions* about the suffering of another against the patient's own subjective experience. The appearance of physical comfort does not necessarily mean that someone has found inner peace. Even in the absence of pain, some patients may feel that life has lost any semblance of meaning or purpose; or as one patient put it, "that breathing has become redundant."

Fortunately, this kind of abject anguish is rare, but there are gradations of suffering that are much more common: people anticipate losing everything they know and love, the severing of all ties to this life, and an unknowable future. Suffering of this nature is ubiquitous and can range from the obviously painful to the silent and unspoken subtleties. Dignity Therapy can be broadly applied, ranging from those who express severe distress to those who express no distress whatsoever. In other words, Dignity Therapy need not be applied only in instances of obvious end-of-life distress and anguish. Rather, it can be used in circumstances where patients feel this might provide them comfort and enhance meaning and purpose in their final months, weeks, or days of life.

Just as we cannot assume to know the nature of someone's suffering, neither can we assume to know who might benefit from Dignity Therapy. This is not to say that every patient will benefit from Dignity Therapy or that every patient should take part. One patient approached for Dignity Therapy responded by saying, "If what you are suggesting will help me get from here to the toilet on my own, I'm interested; if not, feel free to leave any time!" On the other hand, one needs to be broad minded when considering who might benefit from, and who to approach for, a therapeutic trial.

Dignity Therapy aims to instill a sense of meaning and purpose for its participants by providing an effective foil to feeling a burden or a mounting sense of futility, which can emerge when illness and loss become overwhelming. By engaging patients in the telling of their story and having them convey important thoughts, feelings, and wishes, Dignity Therapy helps safeguard and promote a sense of being worthwhile or valued. It is easy to imagine how certain assumptions might preclude some patients from being considered for Dignity Therapy. One might presume, for instance, that certain stories, life experiences, and even personality styles lend themselves better than others to Dignity Therapy. Experience has shown that until we ask, it is impossible to know who might value and in turn benefit from Dignity Therapy. Time and again, Dignity Therapy has shown us that every life is unique, as are the relationships forged, experiences accumulated, and insights revealed. The seemingly "ordinary life" becomes extraordinary when we take the time to look at it closely. As Ralph Waldo Emerson noted, explore a single individual deeply enough and truths about all individuals emerge. It is safe to assume that *every* patient has a story to tell, insights to share, memories or wishes they might want to pass along by means of Dignity Therapy—and the best way to affirm this is simply by asking.

Who Should Be Approached to Take Part in Dignity Therapy?

Eligibility Criterion 1: Anyone Facing Life-Threatening or Life- Limiting Circumstances

Although more patients with cancer than any other disease group have taken part in Dignity Therapy, it has been used successfully in patients with neurodegenerative disorders (such as muscular dystrophy and ALS), end-stage renal disease, end-stage chronic obstructive pulmonary disease, and participants who might best be described as the frail elderly. Conditions that interfere with a patient's ability to communicate can be challenging and, in some instances, may preclude their being able to participate. However, patients with speaking difficulties, such as those seen in later stages of ALS, have taken part in our studies of Dignity Therapy. Creative thinking, patience and ingenuity, the presence of a family member to help facilitate or elaborate some of the responses, and/or the use of a keyboard or similar facilitative communication device can enable patients without a voice to articulate their Dignity Therapy responses. One gentleman, who had had a laryngectomy as a result of head and neck cancer, typed each of his answers using ornate fonts to embellish his responses.

Another issue that is sometimes raised is whether insight and prognostic awareness are important qualifiers for Dignity Therapy. Dignity Therapy does not depend on patients acknowledging or wanting to discuss their impending death. As a general rule of thumb, however, the potency and poignancy of Dignity Therapy seems to intensify as proximity to death shortens and death awareness heightens. Neither of these are prerequisites for participation, and it is certainly not the role of the Dignity Therapist to engage in conversations that disclose new prognostic information. However, patients who are aware of their limited life expectancy approach this generativity-base therapy differently, perhaps more reflectively, and with more urgency and honesty than those who do not anticipate a foreshortened lifespan. The difference is how one faces a final chance versus one of many such chances. Approaching Dignity Therapy as a final opportunity to share memories, thoughts, and reflections provides an existential intensity that might otherwise be lacking.

A nineteen-year-old young man, whose therapeutic options for leukemia were all but depleted, was invited to participate in Dignity Therapy. His home life was rather chaotic, with his father long since gone from the family scene, and his only sibling—a twenty-three-year-old sister—actively rebelling against her strong-willed mother. In spite of his dire medical circumstances, he did not think or speak in terms of his time being limited. Although he was able to respond to many of the Dignity Therapy questions, his answers lacked intensity or urgency. For instance, when asked about advice or wishes to pass along to his sister, he voiced wanting to speak to her "one day" about the importance of going back and completing high school. When asked if he would like to speak to those issues now, he responded by indicating that he would do so at some point, when the time felt right.

Eligibility Criterion 2: The Patient Is Interested in Dignity Therapy and Feels Motivated to Take Part

Motivation to take part in Dignity Therapy is hard to predict. Yet feeling a sense of resonance with this intervention is as good an indicator as any that the choice to take part is right. Therefore, patients should fully understand what they are getting into, including the specific kinds of questions they will be asked. This is important, not only for the purposes of informed consent but also to help patients determine whether Dignity Therapy strikes them as personally meaningful and worthwhile. Taking time to consider the questions that they might encounter in Dignity Therapy also helps patients mentally prepare for the intervention itself. There is nothing to be gained by withholding information about Dignity Therapy from the prospective participant; rather, full disclosure ensures that they are keen to take part and engage in the kind of reflection and personal sharing that this approach entails.

The patient's expressed interest and motivation in Dignity Therapy is a critical test of their suitability for this particular treatment. It is hard to say what typifies patients who select Dignity Therapy, but they often sense that this is a way enhancing meaning and purpose and that it merits investing some of their precious time and energy. Although patients conceive the outcome of Dignity Therapy in various ways, many see it as a way of helping themselves, while also providing benefits to those they love and care about.

Eligibility Criterion 3: To Participate in Dignity Therapy, the Patient, and Therapist and Transcriptionist Must All Speak the Same Language

Although most of the work on Dignity Therapy has taken place in English-speaking countries such as Canada, the United States, England, and Australia, trials have also been carried out, or are ongoing, in Denmark, Portugal, Japan, China, and French-speaking Canada. To conduct Dignity Therapy, it is critical that the therapist, patient, and transcriptionist (see section on editing) all speak the same language. The language the patient wishes the document to be written needs to be determined well before proceeding with Dignity Therapy. The person transcribing the interview and the person editing the transcript must be fluent in the patient's language choice.

Who Should Not Take Part in Dignity Therapy?

Dignity therapy is not a panacea; not everyone needs it nor will everyone necessarily benefit from it. A general truism in medicine is that any therapy with potency can also have adverse effects. This also applies to Dignity Therapy in that good and bad outcomes are possible. To minimize the latter, it is important to think about who should not be approached to take part in Dignity Therapy.

Exclusion Criterion 1: Anyone Who Is Too Ill and Who Is Not Expected to Live More than About Two Weeks Should Not, Under Normal Circumstances, Be Considered for Dignity Therapy

The most common reason that patients decline Dignity Therapy is that they feel too ill. Advanced disease depletes patients of their physical and mental energy. The role of the therapist is to help the patient organize their thoughts, provide cues that will guide their responses, and use techniques that will encourage them to offer additional details, thereby facilitating their responses. Nevertheless, patients still require enough energy and mental wherewithal to embark on this reflective therapeutic intervention. Normally, only patients expected to be alive within a two-week time frame—the time it usually takes to complete the entire intervention—should be offered Dignity Therapy. Failure to complete Dignity Therapy can deny patients the opportunity to fully have their say or can interfere with their seeing and approving their edited generativity document.

There have been a few instances in which patients in our Dignity Therapy studies have started the intervention but have not been able to complete the protocol. Even with careful selection processes, this is bound to happen occasionally. This situation presents the therapist with several challenges that will need to be addressed. For instance, what should happen to an incomplete transcript? Who does it belong to? Whose role is it to facilitate these decisions? Experience has taught us that there is wisdom in asking the patient, at the conclusion of their Dignity Therapy session, how they would like the transcript to be handled, should they feel too ill to attend to it later. We usually say, "If you are feeling too unwell when I return with the edited transcript, do I have your permission to complete it to the best of my ability, and give it to [whomever they have designated as the target recipient]?" The therapist might also seek the patient's permission to approach the intended document recipients for assistance with any editing issues, should they arise. This simple precautionary measure helps avoid an assortment of difficulties and preempts various ethical dilemmas that might otherwise arise.

Occasionally, there may be an exception to the two-week survival criterion, but this takes concerted planning and resources to achieve. Sometimes a patient, in spite of advanced disease and little time left, expresses a strong desire to proceed with Dignity Therapy. If therapy is going to be offered in this circumstance, the entire time frame needs to be reduced substantively. This is possible, although it means that everyone involved in the entire process—the patient, the therapist, and the transcriptionist—need to be invested in this quick turnaround time.

Ms. M. was a forty-nine-year-old woman with advanced lung cancer. At the time of her Dignity Therapy interview, it was apparent that she was profoundly ill and that her life expectancy would likely be days rather than weeks. She had heard about Dignity Therapy from the ward staff and expressed a keen interest in taking part. Widespread lung metastases made it difficult for her to speak. Nevertheless, in little more than faint whispers, she was able to express her love for her young daughter and recount some early memories for her daughter to cherish. This included telling the story of how she chose her daughter's name, based on her own adolescent recollection of a particularly endearing foreign film character.

Given her very tenuous clinical condition, her interview was transcribed and edited overnight and returned the following day. She was moved to tears by the result. A few days later, she died.

Exclusion Criterion 2: One of the Most Important Reasons to Exclude Patients from Dignity Therapy Is Impaired Cognitive Ability, Limiting the Patient's Capacity to Provide Meaningful and Reflective Responses

The importance of cognitive ability cannot be overemphasized. Delirium, cognitive clouding, or cognitive failure is not uncommon among terminally ill patients. In fact, most patients experience an interval of cognitive impairment prior to death. Hence, it is imperative to initiate and complete Dignity Therapy prior to loss of cognitive capacity (see box 2). Patients who are actively psychotic are not good candidates for Dignity Therapy. Pseudodementia, which refers to poverty of thought that can occur with serious depression, should also be screened for, as its consequences are no less distorting than dementia itself. These patients are often overwhelmed by feelings of guilt and self-deprecation. Again, this can result in tainting Dignity Therapy with a false representation of self.

Dr. M. was a seventy-two-year-old retired professor at a local university. During the course of his career, his academic achievements had been considerable. Within his professional community, he was well known and respected for his various scholarly accomplishments. According to his wife, he had also been a good husband and a highly involved and loving father to his two now-grown children. Nevertheless, in his early responses to Dignity Therapy, he seemed unable to recount many of the positive attributes of his career and he portrayed himself as having failed his family by placing work obligations ahead of them. His wife was able to point out that this was inaccurate and reflected a depressive stance that had emerged over the last several weeks of his illness. In view of these cognitive distortions and his relative poverty of thought, it was suggested to Dr. M. that he could try this some other time, when he might be in a better frame of mind to proceed. He readily agreed.

As it turned out, the inclination not to proceed with Dignity Therapy was well founded, given that he died within a few days of our initial contact. Had we proceeded with the interview, Dr. M.'s responses would have painted a picture of a man barely recognizable to his family. While he appeared to have little to say about his personal life and, in fact, implied that he had let his wife and children down in his role as a father and husband, these perceptions ran counter to those of his family.

The consequences of failing to identify this type of cognitive impairment or distortion can be devastating. Although the majority of patients and their families who have taken part in Dignity Therapy felt highly satisfied with the intervention, the exceptions have been in instances in which cognitive limitations were not detected prior to, or during, the therapy itself. This is most unfortunate, in that it results in a generativity document that is, as one dissatisfied family described, "a distortion of who they really were."

Creating a distorted representation of the patient is perhaps the most significant toxicity that can emerge from Dignity Therapy. Sadly, there is usually little opportunity to undo this harm prior to the further deterioration and death of the patient. Safeguards in the editing process and the terms of consent can help contain this harm and are described later. In the few instances when this occurred, the family member recipient of the generativity document held back the document rather than the usual sharing among others close to the patient.

Step 2. Once eligibility has been determined, Dignity Therapy can be formally introduced to the patient and family.

Dignity Therapy is a well-researched intervention that can enhance end-of-life experience for people dealing with life-limiting medical conditions. Being offered Dignity Therapy does not imply mental illness or even that the patient is not coping well. In fact, many patients who participate in Dignity Therapy clinical trials indicate that although they thought they were coping adequately, Dignity Therapy provides important therapeutic benefits. To some extent, the choice of wording used to introduce Dignity Therapy will depend upon the patient's degree of insight and openness in talking about their medical circumstances. Clinicians should never lose sight of the importance of communication skills in palliative care. Exquisite communication goes hand in hand with exquisite listening. The therapist should never assume full prognostic awareness and must, therefore, listen carefully to how the patient describes his or her medical condition. It is a mistake to assume that terms such as "palliative," "terminal," or "death and dying" are emotionally benign when introducing Dignity Therapy without some indication from the patient to that effect. Stating that Dignity Therapy is an intervention for patients who are near the end of life or who are terminally ill is a poor way to begin.

A Typical Dignity Therapy Introduction

Your doctor/nurse tells me that you are interested in Dignity Therapy. I thought I would stop by and tell you a little bit about it and answer any questions you might have. Dignity Therapy is a talking therapy that has been specially designed to help people who are living with significant medical challenges. There have been several studies done on Dignity Therapy and the results indicate that it can help many people cope, improve how they feel about themselves and their circumstances, and even improve their quality of life. It can also have benefits for their family members. Dignity Therapy usually only takes one session, sometimes two. It gives people a chance to talk about things that are most important to them, things that they want to share with those they are closest to and things that they feel they need and want to say. These conversations are audio recorded, transcribed, and edited. The final product is a type-written document or paper, which is returned to you. Most people find the experience very meaningful and find comfort in knowing that the document is for them to keep and something they can share with people they care about.

This example provides a sense of the information we provide when introducing Dignity Therapy (see Step 3 box). The tone should be kept informal and the format conversational.

Step 3. Once Dignity Therapy has been introduced, answer any questions that the patient might have.

Patients may have several questions. Each question must be acknowledged and appropriately addressed. Offer responses that foster a sense of comfort and trust.

Some Common Questions and Responses

1. Why do you think Dignity Therapy works?

Dignity Therapy is based on research that shows that many people who are quite ill feel that who they are, and the things that they used to do that made them feel like themselves and feel useful, can start to fade. These feelings will vary from person to person and may even fluctuate at any given time. Being sick, however, can get in the way of people feeling like themselves. Dignity Therapy is meant to help people, especially those who are feeling particularly unwell, maintain the sense that they still have something important to do. Dignity Therapy gives people a chance to talk about important things. Just as compelling, it gives people a chance to look after people they care about by creating a deeply personal document that they can share. It also gives people a feeling that, no matter what happens, the words that they share will be kept safe and can't be touched by their illness.

2. What sort of questions will I need to answer?

Actually, there won't be any questions that you must answer. This is your therapy and the document that we create will belong to you. Therefore, I want you to feel free to talk about only things that you want to talk about; if I happen to ask you something that you'd rather not talk about, we will simply move on.

3. What kinds of questions will you ask me?

I have an outline of questions that covers topics such as: what you would like loved ones to know about you or specific words or thoughts that you would like to take an opportunity to say. In fact, I plan on leaving you a copy of the question outline so that you can read it over and give some thought about if or how you would like to answer some or all of the questions. This will also give you a chance to think about whether there is something missing from these questions that you would like to talk about.

Occasionally, patients will have a clear notion of the kinds of things they would like to say or the issues they would like to address. This should be encouraged. For example, some patients may wish to reflect on their personal life histories and early development. Others may want to use Dignity Therapy as a way of leaving letters for their children or future generations. Patients who express particular content preferences should be supported to do so by structuring the sessions accordingly. If the patient feels that they need to leave behind a coveted family recipe, the secret to their business success, an apology for past failings, or life lessons to guide their children in the years ahead, then the therapy should be constructed around those stated objectives.

For the most part, patients who agree to participate in Dignity Therapy do not have particular content in mind. For most patients, Dignity Therapy facilitates the wish to tell important elements of their life story and have it remembered. For some patients, this will consist of a brief overview of their history, while others will focus on particular chapters or events that they view as most memorable, formative, or important. Some patients see other clear tasks they would like therapy to facilitate or accomplish. For example, one sad elderly gentleman with a long history of alcohol abuse used his therapy as an opportunity to wish his children and grandchildren "a better life than I had." He stated that he realized it was "too late" to make amends to his children, but wanted his grandchildren to know the truth about him, "so they can choose a better way than I did." Dignity Therapy sessions are structured such that patients can either spontaneously offer important content or use the question protocol to reflect on specific content areas.

4. What if I get started and I just don't know what to say or how to continue?

That's part of my job and that's part of what makes Dignity Therapy possible. I will be here to help you make this work. I will try and think of all the right questions and try to give you all the cues and encouragement you need to get your story told. Dignity Therapy has now been done with hundreds if not thousands of patients around the world, most of whom were quite ill at the time they took part. We have become quite skilled at helping people tell their story. We know when you might need some guidance and direction in order to complete your Dignity Therapy. To make this as comfortable for you as possible, Dignity Therapy lets you add or change anything you like before the process is considered complete.

Patients near the end of life invariably experience diminished energy, which is often physical, emotional, and even cognitive. It is critical that patients participating in Dignity Therapy are cognitively able to respond in ways that will be meaningful to themselves and their families. Due to energy limitations, most patients need help. In our experience, patients are more than willing to be guided through the process. In most instances, responses to the questions are easily elicited, but it is up to the therapist to propel the intervention for patients who lack energy. It is also the therapist's responsibility to insert prompts, point out possible connections, and inject energy into the sessions in order to facilitate rich and meaningful responses (see chapter 5).

5. What if I get tired or just start feeling too unwell to continue?

This is your therapy and we aren't going to do anything that you don't want done. If you are tired or need a break, just say the word, and we will stop. I will ask you periodically if you need or want to take a break; also, depending entirely on your energy, I'll be sure not to go any longer than 45 minutes to an hour at most. I have seen people get absorbed and lose themselves in the process. Not everyone, but some people who start out feeling tired actually find the process engaging and even energizing.

Mr. J. was a seventy-year-old retired teacher with advanced colorectal cancer. He had previously agreed to take part in Dignity Therapy, but on the day of his scheduled session he felt "too sick and too tired" to concentrate. He was told that the session could be rescheduled and that the timing needed to suit him. However, once he spotted the tape recorder, he suggested "we try." With the recording started, Mr. J. sat up in bed and for the next full hour, with very little prompting, recounted his life story, lessons learned, and wishes to be conveyed to his wife, children, and grandchildren.

Similar experiences have been noted by colleagues doing Dignity Therapy in Australia and the United States. Keep in mind that feeling energized by Dignity Therapy does not occur in every instance, and always respect the patient's readiness to proceed.

6. Why does it have to be audio recorded; what if I don't feel comfortable with the tape recorder?

It is not at all unusual for people to feel a bit uncomfortable with the tape recorder at the beginning of Dignity Therapy. I can promise you that within a few minutes into the session, you are likely to forget about the tape recorder entirely. The recording is important for us to be able to transcribe the conversation and then use the transcript to create a document, which you can share with the important people in your life.

Some clinicians may question the importance of the recording. However, it is important to bear in mind the research underpinnings of Dignity Therapy. Recall that based on our studies of terminally ill patients, we developed the Model of Dignity in the Terminally Ill or the Dignity Model.[1,2] The Dignity Model, derived from data of patients in their final weeks to months of life, provided information about critical factors that can support or undermine dignity in the context of approaching death. One major theme that emerged from our analysis was the Dignity-Conserving Repertoire, referring to various psychological and spiritual issues that can shape the experience of living with an advanced, life-threatening, or life-limiting illness. Within this theme emerged the subtheme generativity/legacy. Generativity/legacy refers to the idea that something about who we are or who we have been in this life will outlast us, for the benefit of those left behind. The audio recording of the Dignity Therapy session enables the transcription, which in turn, forms the basis of the generativity document. In this way, Dignity Therapy provides the patient with something quite profound—the ability to have their words transcend death itself.

The idea of nonexistence is impossible for anyone to fully grasp. Each of us wants to believe that a part of who we are will carry on beyond the event of our death, at the very least in the collective memory of those whose lives we have touched. For some, this sense of generativity/legacy will be achieved through children or grandchildren. For others, it may consist of works or accomplishments that will outlive them. For patients who participate in Dignity Therapy, the generativity document can provide tangible and lasting testimony of important thoughts and memories, forever preserved for those they will soon leave behind. As one fifty-eight-year-old woman with metastatic breast cancer said after completing Dignity Therapy one week before her death, "I may not be a famous person, and not many people will remember my name, but my sons will have this [holding the edited document]."

Some clinicians have also raised the possibility of other recording options, such as providing the patient an audio recording or a video recording. The written transcript, however, has several advantages over other media. It disconnects the patient's words from a voice or physical image that may be encumbered by advancing illness. In spite of sickness, words can maintain their power and poignancy without the distraction of how someone looks or sounds.

A patient with end-stage breast cancer arrived by wheelchair to her outpatient Dignity Therapy appointment. Despite her spinal metastases, neck brace, and generalized fatigue, she was able to tell a wonderful and moving story of her difficult childhood, a conflicted relationship with her mother, and rather stormy connections with her own children. In spite of these issues, her responses were a testament of undying love and affection for her family. At the end, when asked if she might have preferred to have her session video recorded, she stated: "this isn't how I look; this is how a woman dying from breast cancer looks!" Although her appearance bore all the markings of someone with advanced disease, her transcribed words were strong and vibrant.

The following example illustrates the emotional rawness that can be conveyed within an unedited Dignity Therapy audio recording.

Several years ago, I was able to meet with the husband of a Dignity Therapy participant about one year after his wife's death. He had been one of the very few people who asked not only to receive the edited generativity document but also the actual Dignity Therapy audio recording. There was no ethical challenge in doing so, since the two of them had done Dignity Therapy together. His wife had been a remarkable woman, who died from complications of metastatic lung cancer. At the time of her therapy, she was so short of breath that speaking to any extent had become a real strain. Between the two of them, however—completing thoughts and sentences for one another—they were able to create a beautiful generativity document.

Meeting one year later brought back memories of that earlier, moving encounter, along with the chance to hear him compare the experience of receiving the generativity document and the unedited audio recording. His response was remarkable. He told me that, "no one" other than he and his son, would ever be told of the tape's existence. "It is simply too raw and too painful to listen to," he explained. On the other hand, "everyone" had a copy of the generativity document, including friends and family. Unlike the audio recording, the generativity document was, and continued to be, a source of comfort.

Because of ease with which words can be edited, using the written transcript as the mode of generativity can enhance the flow of the final generativity document.

Ms. L. was a fifty-five-year-old woman with advanced colorectal cancer. Her Dignity Therapy was marked by frequent interruptions, either to attend to her colostomy bag or simply to find a more comfortable position. These interruptions and occasional distracted thoughts were nowhere to be found in her powerful, final, edited generativity document. Her story detailed a life that began in poverty and was marked by early childhood neglect and abuse. In her early twenties, destitute, alone, and with little to show for her life, she was taken in by a nun "who believed in" her. She credited this relationship with "turning everything around" and enabling her to go on to become a successful health care provider and beloved educator.

Unlike an audio or video recording, a transcript can be easily edited. Words, phrases, or entire passages can be omitted or later added to the transcript (see chapter 5). The final result provides a document that patients can feel proud and confident of, in that it captures what they want to say and how they want it said. Ms. L. wanted "everyone" to have a copy of her transcript—her health care providers, her friends, and her family—so all would know what she went through and the potential that each of us holds within.

7. What if I just don't get it out right? What if I forget to mention something important? Or what if I say something, and don't like the way it sounds? This sounds like an important document, and I'd like to get it perfect. What if I don't get it perfect?

This is where my role as a therapist is important, as is the audio recording. My commitment to you is to use all of my skills and energy to try and make this document the best that it can be. Even though you may not be feeling well, I can help you. Also remember that the transcript will be edited. I will have the first take at this, and then I will read everything to you to be sure that it meets with your approval. If there is something we've missed, we can add it; if there is something there that you don't like, we can fix or even delete it. I will help you correct even the tiniest errors. At the end of this process, I want you to feel comfortable with what you have done. Hundreds of patients have done this and, almost without exception they have been very pleased with the results.

The patient can be reassured that because of the careful editing process, even the most minor of clarifications can be made, as well as the larger issues taken care of, such as chronological corrections and major additions or deletions, prior to declaring the process complete. (More detail about editing the transcript is offered in chapter 5.)

A professor of English Literature decided to undertake Dignity Therapy about two weeks prior to his death. While he had taken great pride in his work life and scholastic accomplishments, nothing compared with the importance he placed on his family, including his wife, children, and grandchildren. He used his Dignity Therapy to remind his grandchildren to always love and respect their mother and father, and to love themselves. Although an atypical request, he felt that he wanted slightly different versions of the generativity document going to his family than the one he planned on sharing with his closest friends. With some modest modifications, these two versions were provided to him to share with others as he saw fit.

8. Is Dignity Therapy just for patients who are dying, and is that why you are offering it to me? (This is not a question I ever recall being asked, but it may come as the uptake of Dignity Therapy increases)

Dignity Therapy was originally developed for people in palliative care; that is, for people nearing their end of life. However, Dignity Therapy has been applied to many people outside of palliative care, including those facing various significant health problems or even some of the challenges of growing older. I can't predict what course your illness or condition will follow. But it seems whether people are close to the end or somewhere well before it, talking about issues that come up in Dignity Therapy usually brings people comfort.

9. How do I know that Dignity Therapy is right for me? (Variations of this question include, I don't have a particularly special story to tell; my life wasn't very interesting.)

Dignity Therapy has been done with people from all walks of life and in various countries around the world. Based on extensive experience, what we have found makes any story special is that it belongs to the teller. No two lives are the same and no two stories are the same. Even lives that patients describe as "ordinary" or "uninteresting" invariably are unique; they are stories that are told by the only ones who are personally able to tell them. Doctors, lawyers, farmers, homemakers, homesteaders, artists, factory workers, journalists, business moguls—there is no easy way of characterizing the kinds of people who find Dignity Therapy helpful. If the idea of Dignity Therapy sounds appealing and meaningful, you should probably try it.

Mrs. S. was a sixty-nine-year-old woman who, fifteen years earlier, had immigrated to Canada with her husband and young children from Eastern Europe. She described her life as having been joyful. She loved being a mother and loved the many opportunities that moving to Canada had opened up to her and her family. With considerable persistence, she had learned English, obtained her drivers license, and gone back to school. During the course of her Dignity Therapy, which she undertook while in palliative care for an advance malignancy, she shared this reflection: "I haven't done anything in great or marvelous ways, but just the small things that you do are important." In anticipation of her own death, she used Dignity Therapy as an opportunity to try to console her family: "I have to go eventually, but I don't want to . . . leave you in despair. I know that you are going to make it without me. . . . It will be okay."

10. What if I think I'm doing fine without Dignity Therapy; why should I bother?

Not everyone needs or will want Dignity Therapy. However, we have offered it to people who feel distressed and others who feel they have been managing well. Even for the latter group, Dignity Therapy has been reported by most to be helpful, to heighten a sense of meaning and purpose, and to improve quality of life. Ultimately, you should be guided by what feels best for you.

11. Do I have to do Dignity Therapy on my own? Is it OK to have someone with me during the interview?

Dignity Therapy can be done on your own or with someone by your side. Whichever choice works best for you will probably work best for the therapy. Some people do it on their own because it feels more private and more comfortable, making it easier to share personal thoughts, feelings, and recollections. You might feel less restricted in what you say if you don't have to take into account the needs of a friend or family member who may be looking for certain content to be included in your document. If you think you might feel uncomfortable or as though you have to "perform" for someone else, then you should probably consider doing Dignity Therapy on your own. That way, you won't have to worry how someone else might feel, or what they might be thinking during the course of the therapy.

On the other hand, some people feel more comfortable and safer having a friend or family member with them. If this person knows you well, he or she might be able to offer help in identifying directions that the therapy can move into. Keep in mind that there is no right or wrong answer to this question; it is simply a matter of what feels best for you.

Step 4. After all the patient's questions have been answered, offer him or her a copy of the basic Dignity Therapy question protocol.

Giving patients a copy of the Dignity Therapy question protocol serves a variety of purposes (see box 4). It demystifies the process by providing patients a much clearer idea of what the therapy entails. As important, it allows patients time to reflect on the questions and deliberate on how they might wish to respond. After all, if the generativity document is meant to be part of his or her legacy, it is to the patient's and therapist's great advantage if some thought has been given to how these questions might be answered. Finally, being familiar with the question protocol in advance gives patients an opportunity to consider whether there are areas or issues they might wish to broach, which are not part of the therapy question protocol. In our experience, offering patients a copy of these questions when Dignity Therapy is being introduced works well. Occasionally, patients will have a clear sense of how to shape their Dignity Therapy. Taking control of the content in this way, to the extent they are able, should be encouraged. One woman in her mid-sixties with advanced lung cancer felt that Dignity Therapy was an ideal opportunity to say things to her children and grandchildren so they might benefit from the wisdom of her insights and warmth of her blessings.

Most patients, at least initially, do not offer particular content preferences. Instead, they defer to the expertise and judgment of the therapist until they have a better sense of the interview and the direction they wish to take it. For those patients, the interview protocol will form the structural basis of their Dignity Therapy. This protocol, and the specific questions it contains, is based on the Model of Dignity in the Terminally Ill[1] (see chapter 1). It is important for the therapist to understand that the Dignity Therapy questions are not arbitrary or haphazard. They have been designed to elicit responses and address subject areas that might invoke a sense of meaning and purpose, and connect people to memories and thoughts that will resonate most closely with their core sense of self.

THE DIGNITY THERAPY QUESTION PROTOCOL

The Dignity Therapy Question Protocol is comprised of questions that are based on the Dignity Model (see Step 5 box). Each question is meant to elicit some aspect of personhood, provide an opportunity for affirmation, or help the participant reconnect with elements of self that were, or perhaps still remain, meaningful or valued. As described in the next chapter, there is far more to delivering Dignity Therapy than simply posing each of these questions in turn. Nevertheless, they are the framework for Dignity Therapy and vital for the delivery of this unique therapeutic intervention.

- Tell me a little about your life history; particularly the parts that you either remember most or think are the most important.
- When did you feel most alive?
- Are there particular things that you would want your family to know about you, and are there particular things you would want them to remember?
- What are the most important roles you have played in your life (e.g., family roles, vocational roles, community service roles)? Why were they so important to you, and what do you think you accomplished within those roles?
- What are your most important accomplishments, and what do you feel most proud of or take most pride in?
- Are there particular things that you feel need to be said to your loved ones or things that you would want to take the time to say once again?
- What are your hopes and dreams for your loved ones?
- What have you learned about life that you would want to pass along to others? What advice or words of guidance would you wish to pass along to your [son, daughter, husband, wife, parents, other(s)]?
- Are there important words, or perhaps even instructions, you would like to offer your family?
- In creating this permanent record, are there other things that you would like included?

These questions were designed to target issues related most closely to the patient's sense of personhood, essence, or core self. Notice that the questions address and, in turn, invite the patient to discuss aspects of life that are, or were, most important, most memorable, and most worthy of being remembered. By engaging in a dialogue in which these issues are front and center, patients may feel that their core self is being acknowledged, thus bolstering in patients a sense of meaning, purpose, and dignity. These questions are meant to act as a guide for therapists providing Dignity Therapy. They are not intended to be rigid or prescriptive or in any way to limit the scope of Dignity Therapy. In fact, the therapist not only has the latitude, but also the responsibility, to explore these and other questions that arise during the course of the session. The therapist must skilfully guide the flow of the interview based on the patient's interest and individual responses. Hence it is critical that the therapist assume a facilitative role.

Step 5. Once the patient has agreed to take part, collect basic demographic information. This will help guide the content of the upcoming Dignity Therapy interview.

Baseline information before proceeding with Dignity Therapy should include the patients' name and how they would like to be addressed; their age, marital status, who they live with and where, and whether or not they have children or grandchildren (including their names and ages). It is also helpful to ask about their vocation and current employment status. The therapist will also want to know how long the patients have been sick, the nature of their illness, and how they understand the gravity of their condition. This information provides a metaphorical frame within which the Dignity Therapy interview paints the detailed picture (see Step 6 box). This frame also prevents the possibility of inadvertently neglecting some basic or formative aspect of the patients' life (e.g., a child, a partner, or some other core facet of self).

Step 6. Arrange an appointment with the patient (with or without a friend, family member, or loved one) to conduct the Dignity Therapy interview.

The session is usually scheduled to take place within the shortest feasible time frame after the introductory meeting has taken place, questions have been answered, and the patient has consented to participate. This can be within one to ideally no more than three days. Timely follow-up throughout Dignity Therapy is important and reinforces an ethos of immediacy. This conveys a tangible message—that what the patient has to say is important and that the therapist will move quickly to capture the patient's all-important thoughts and words. Flexibility during this time frame, however, should be based on the individual patient's needs and wishes.

Dignity Therapy, like any talking therapy, should take place where the patient is as comfortable as possible. Thus far, these sessions have been held almost equally between institutional settings (palliative care units, personal care homes, acute care wards) and in patients' homes. Privacy, of course, is important, in that it gives people permission to give voice to various matters that they might consider personal and intended only for a select few. However, advanced illness can sometimes challenge privacy, necessitating creativity and flexibility. Drawing a bed curtain, finding seating for the therapist and Dignity Therapy participants, scheduling the session so as not to disrupt care needs, reducing ambient noise (TV, radio)—all of these measures help create an intimate milieu within which Dignity Therapy can successfully take place. Having made the necessary preparations, it is time to get started.

REFERENCES

1. Chochinov HM, Hack T, McClement S, Kristjanson L, Harlos M. Dignity in the terminally ill: a developing empirical model. *Soc Sci Med.* 2002;54(3):433–443.
2. Chochinov HM. Dignity-conserving care—a new model for palliative care: helping the patient feel valued. *JAMA.* 2002;287(17):2253–2260.
3. Chochinov HM, Hack T, Hassard T, Kristjanson LJ, McClement S, Harlos M. Dignity and psychotherapeutic considerations in end-of-life care. *J Palliat Care.* 2004;20(3):134–142.
4. Chochinov HM. Dying, dignity, and new horizons in palliative end-of-life care. *CA Cancer J Clin.* 2006;56(2):84–103.
5. McClement SE, Chochinov HM, Hack TF, Kristjanson LJ, Harlos M. Dignity-conserving care: application of research findings to practice. *Int J Palliat Nurs.* 2004;10(4):173–179.

4

DOING DIGNITY THERAPY

Care more particularly for the individual patient than for the special features of the disease.
—William Osler

Thus far, we have reviewed the importance of dignity as a clinically meaningful construct and provided an overview of how empirical research addressing dignity toward the end of life led to the development of Dignity Therapy.[1-4] Based on this foundation, chapter 3 provided detailed, step-by-step instructions on how to identify potential Dignity Therapy participants and to arrange the actual Dignity Therapy session. Chapter 4 moves beyond these preparatory steps, taking us to the heart of the matter, that is, actually doing Dignity Therapy.

By the time the therapist and patient arrive together for the Dignity Therapy session, several things should have already been accomplished:

- Dignity Therapy has been explained to the patient, and he or she has agreed to take part.
- The patient has been given a copy of the Dignity Therapy question protocol, which provides an opportunity to reflect on possible content for the generativity document. There is nothing to be gained by withholding this information; if anything, being more aware of the protocol will set patients' minds at ease and help them to be better prepared.
- The patient has determined who, within their family or broad social network, would be the most appropriate recipient(s) of this important document.
- The patient has decided whether to do Dignity Therapy alone or accompanied by a friend or family member.

- The therapist has established the "frame" for the patient's Dignity Therapy, that is, their name and how they wish to be addressed, age, marital status, names and ages of significant others (such as children, grandchildren), vocation, what illness they have and what they understand of their condition.
- I recall asking a patient, as part of the framing exercise, what he hoped to accomplish by doing Dignity Therapy. He explained that he had made a lot of mistakes in his life. He felt especially guilty that, following his leaving his first marriage for another woman, he had been less than available to his children. In spite of the success and longevity of that relationship, he felt he owed his children an explanation and an apology. Knowing this before hand made it easy to accommodate him being able to address these key issues within the course of his Dignity Therapy.

SETTING UP THE DIGNITY THERAPY SESSION

Answering Remaining Questions

Upon arriving to the Dignity Therapy session, therapists should offer to review things once more. It is not unusual for patients to have questions, considering that attentional abilities may be limited when people are very ill. All aspects of the protocol that are unclear to the patient should be explained, with no questions left unanswered. A good way to summarize Dignity Therapy is to explain that it has two primary components. One component of Dignity Therapy consists of a guided conversation between the patient and therapist, addressing issues that the patient deems most important, such as elements of their history, lessons learned, hopes and wishes to convey, or blessings to bestow. The second component of Dignity Therapy consists of creating a very special document. This document will be a record of their therapy session, later edited by the therapist, in order to clearly capture the essence of the patient's responses. Patients will be provided with the edited record, or generativity document, to keep or to share with anyone they wish. Identifying a potential recipient(s) of the document prior to or during the therapy session can make referring to certain people within the interview more tangible, and allows patients to shape their responses with particular individuals in mind. This usually makes for a more effective and meaningful document, as opposed to one that can seem generic, when the patient has no particular recipient in mind.

Arranging the Therapeutic Setting

The setting for Dignity Therapy will have been determined at the conclusion of the initial meeting. At the time of the actual Dignity Therapy session, try to maximize privacy and comfort as much as possible. This is usually easier to accomplish in the patient's home than in a hospital or institutional setting. However, effort and creativity can usually establish an appropriate milieu, even in the middle of a busy hospital ward. Staff can be advised when Dignity Therapy is scheduled and the timing of rounds and care routines can be mutually accommodated so that no one is unduly inconvenienced. As is the case with any other important treatment modality, scheduling challenges can usually be overcome.

In the one-hour interval during which the Dignity Therapy interview is usually completed, visitors can be restricted, and the television or radio turned off, so as to minimize distractions. In some instances, particularly if the patient is not in a private room, a meeting room or office might be used or, if necessary, the curtains drawn around the patient's bed. The therapist should be in close enough proximity to the patient, so that both can easily speak to, see, and hear one other. This reduces the need to speak loudly and establishes a sense of intimacy and privacy. If the patient has decided to have a friend or family member be part of the therapy, this person should be seated next to the patient, opposite the therapist. That is, if the therapist is to the right of the patient, the friend or family member can be seated on the patient's left. Besides its functional advantages, this physical placement is also meant to underscore the message that the therapist's primary task is to speak with the patient, and that the family or friend is there in a supportive and facilitative capacity. Prior to beginning the Dignity Therapy session, ensure that the patient is as comfortable as possible, is offered something to drink, and that facial tissue is on hand.

Using an Audio Recorder

Use a good quality audio recorder and, although it may seem a small detail, test it to ensure that it is working properly. Patients are in a tenuous state of health, so there may be no second chance if the recorder malfunctions. Patients' voices will often be soft and the recording environment less than ideal. Because the interview will be transcribed verbatim, it is important to position the microphone as close to the patient as possible to ensure a clear and audible recording.

Some patients may feel trepidation about committing their thoughts to words, knowing that whatever they say will be recorded. To allay their anxiety, remind patients that because the conversation is being recorded and then transcribed, any changes whatsoever can be made to the transcript; anything can be added, deleted, or, should they so choose, the entire manuscript can be discarded (of all of patients who have done Dignity Therapy, none have opted for that particular option). Also remind patients that because the conversation is being recorded, the manuscript can be edited so that chronological inconsistencies, interruptions, and false starts can all be eliminated. Patients are invariably comforted knowing that the therapist will take on much of the responsibility to transform the recorded conversation into a final generativity document, which meets with their approval.

Family or Friend Participant

The actual Dignity Therapy session is likely to be the first time the therapist will meet whoever the patient may have asked to join them. Be mindful and sensitive to the likelihood that that person will also have some questions or matters they wish to clarify. Openly and honestly answering all questions will provide the patient and family the comfort, confidence, and sense of safety that will make it easier for them to proceed.

Just before the audio recorder is turned on, remind the patient that the first question you will ask them will be about specific recollections or memories that they would like to include in their document. Unless they have any further questions, the audio recorder can be started and Dignity Therapy can begin. "Tell me a little about your life history, particularly the parts that you either remember most or think are the most important."

THE ROLE OF THE DIGNITY THERAPIST

There is a great deal more to Dignity Therapy than simply reading the question protocol to patients and passively awaiting their responses. While some patients may not require much guidance or explicit direction, others may feel completely overwhelmed or even paralyzed, trying to summarize the essence of who they are, or articulating what they want said. The therapist's role in Dignity Therapy is therefore critical.

> At all times, the therapist must be a highly engaged, active listener.

Throughout the course of Dignity Therapy, therapists must pay careful attention to everything that is happening between themselves and their patients, including what is said, how it is said, and even what the subtle nonverbal cues may be saying. Metaphorically, the process is akin to accompanying someone on a quest, who is uncertain what path to follow. The role of the therapist, through active listening, is to ensure that they do not get lost and that they are successful in reaching their destination. This means being ever vigilant, ever on the lookout for where responses might be leading them, tracking the flow of the interview, and anticipating when problems might arise. The tension of allowing patients to move independently and yet knowing when to guide them, even actively redirect them, is the essence of active listening and facilitation in Dignity Therapy. It is simply not possible to accomplish this task without full attention and complete engagement.

At the outset of his Dignity Therapy, an elderly man with advanced cancer seemed rather disengaged as he shared some memories of adolescence. The moment he mentioned music, he became energized and more attentive. Being sensitive to this shift in tone, the therapist asked him about his relationship with music. This moved the patient to sharing how music had shaped his life, had been a part of many wonderful relationships, and was a permanent fixture in his repertoire of lifetime passions.

Sometimes the patient's cues can be very subtle; however, the active and engaged therapist will be ever vigilant, taking note of them when they arise.

An octogenarian recounted the members of his extensive, but now largely deceased (other than one brother) family of origin. He began by mentioning that his mother and father were "beautiful people" but quickly moved on to listing his brother and sisters, with little information, other than their names and birth order. The therapist said, "Now you mentioned that you had beautiful parents— can you fill that in a little bit for me; in what way were they beautiful?" This led to tender memories, in which he recalled how his mother doted on all her many children and how they were the center of her universe.

> At all times, for all patients, and in all circumstances, the therapist must assume a dignity-affirming stance.

A dignity-affirming stance speaks to the therapist's ability to make patients feel respected and valued throughout the therapeutic process. The therapist needs to be a caring *active listener,* who is comfortable with existential issues, silences, and emotions ranging from joy to sorrow. By means of compassionate engagement, the therapy itself—aside from the product it yields—should make patients feel that who they are and the words they speak are important, in fact, exquisitely so. This ethos of caring and support within a relational milieu that is accepting and nonjudgmental is fundamental to the success of Dignity Therapy. Dignity Therapy is meant to enhance care tenor (described in the Dignity Model).[1,2] This therapeutic stance is meant to convey respect for who the patient is and was, for their thoughts and feelings, and of course for their words—the very words that will be used to construct their generativity document.

It is not enough, however, to act empathic, caring and interested; to conduct Dignity Therapy, those feelings must be authentic. The essence of a dignity-affirming stance is to understand that patients look to the therapist for affirmation and some indication of their inherent worth. Therapists must think of themselves akin to a mirror into which patients gaze for a reflection that captures the essence of who they are and not simply "what illness they have." This is a powerful and empowering metaphor, which confers tremendous therapeutic opportunity to anyone with patient contact. Without authentic engagement and genuine investment, Dignity Therapy will feel vacant and, not surprisingly, will fall short of its therapeutic mark.

One elderly woman took part in Dignity Therapy about a month before her death. She thought of herself and her life as being quite ordinary. With the therapist's encouragement and "in-the-moment" affirmation of the importance of her story, the patient concluded: "Well, I guess everybody in their lifetime would like to leave some kind of legacy. And I suppose for me it's probably been that I don't feel like I've accomplished any tremendous things in my life. It's all been very ordinary stuff. Not like some people who have done wonders in the world, and everybody knows their name. I guess these are things that you would like to be known for, but you won't be in my case. I led an ordinary enough life, but I think I've left good memories and feelings. I have a good reputation and integrity—that will be what I'm leaving. And hopefully that will be enough. I think that's pretty well all I can say about me, because I have never been a flashy person, and I don't think I ever will be. I guess even as plain as it may be, there's always something that you contributed, sometimes without even knowing it. I've enjoyed doing this, and I think what I would do is probably give a copy of this to each of my children.

> Provide the necessary structure and guidance to help the patient construct his or her generativity document.

In Dignity Therapy, the therapist must be prepared to take an active role. The therapist must be able to engage and guide the patient in this meaning-enhancing therapy. Patients who are very ill and moving toward the end of their lives generally lack the energy and initiative to perfectly organize or sequence their responses. For patients to readily move through Dignity Therapy, the therapist needs to follow their leads, while at the same time providing structure that enables them to easily follow sequences, provide elaboration, or make logical connections. There should be a high degree of collaboration between the therapist and the patient to ensure that the patient feels engaged, encouraged, and nurtured.

> Place meaningful, easy to follow "dots!"

One way of thinking about the role of the therapist is to recall the child's game of "draw by numbers." Numbered dots are connected in sequence to help even the least skilled artist make simple or complex shapes. Without the dots to guide the drawing, the task for most would be difficult, if not impossible. Similarly, the role of the Dignity Therapist is to supply patients with the necessary "dots" in order to help them *draw* their own generativity or legacy document. Patients who undertake Dignity Therapy often have little time left to live and little energy to spare. Although the completion of a life narrative could very well heighten their sense of meaning or purpose, most patients simply cannot do this on their own. However, by skillfully supplying the appropriate "dots," the Dignity Therapist can facilitate the completion of a meaningful generativity document.

Open-ended questions often provide an initial starting point, with the interview generally beginning with the question, "Tell me a little about your life history, particularly the parts that you either remember most, or think are the most important." One elderly gentleman began his response to this question by stating, "The first time I saw my wife, I liked her. We got married and have been married until now." He did not volunteer further detail, and yet it was obvious to the therapist that there was a great deal more to be said. Eliciting detail, laying the "next dot" so that the patient can continue the story, is a critical task for the therapist. In this instance, the following question was asked: "You said when you first saw her, you liked her. Do you remember what you liked?" This led to wonderful reminiscence of having first spotted his future wife at a community hall dance those many years ago, along with recollections of their courtship and eventual marriage. Thus, while the initial question was very broad in scope, the follow-up question moved the patient to become much more specific and much more detailed.

Soon, however, the patient found himself feeling that there was "little more to say." To elicit further detail and help the patient move out of feeling stuck, the therapist offered the following question: "Many events took place between the time you married and now. Are there particular memories or episodes along the way that you want to talk about, or think important to mention?" Notice that the wording does not solicit, nor require, a detailed chronological recounting of the patient's history. Such a pedantic, biographical approach would be untenable; patients would quickly become depleted and the intervention itself cumbersome and impractical. Rather than trying to achieve a sense of historical completeness, questions should elicit focused detail—that is, detail about circumscribed life events or experiences. The patient responded by offering the fact that he "never had a problem with my children." Although he may indeed not have wished, or needed, to say anything further on this issue, this assumption was tested by offering this question: "Are there some special memories of your children growing up that you would like to talk about?" This question elicited detailed information regarding his children, their individual respective milestones, and the feelings and special memories he held for each of them.

Sometimes "placing the dots" requires an ability to be creative, spontaneous, and to follow the patient's cues. For example, one aboriginal woman with advanced colorectal cancer indicated that her spiritual animal was the turtle. The therapist decided to ask about how this came about and its significance. As a result, the patient revealed some deeply held personal values, and how her culture and the history of her people shaped her sense of place in the world. Spontaneous questioning of this kind can facilitate a meaningful, rich, and textured narrative. This will heighten the patient's sense of purpose, meaning, and dignity, which in turn, can result in a generativity document that holds great significance for family and loved ones.

> Sit side-by-side with the patient, looking through a metaphorical photo album.

Another way of eliciting detail is to say to patients, "Imagine that you and I are looking through a photo-album of your life. Tell me, in as much detail as you can, about some of the pictures we might see." This is a simple but yet very effective metaphor to apply in Dignity Therapy. Photographs are tangible artifacts of the moments they capture. In Dignity Therapy, patients, in effect, are invited to scan a mental photo album, selecting those images that happen to resonate as important or memorable. Asking about the people, places or events documented in these mental pictures often jogs the patient's memory and brings out further meaningful material for their generativity document. Having patients scan the album provides breadth; delving into the details of the individual pictures offers depth. It is this depth, referring to the detail of a particular "photograph," which makes the responses personal and unique. Using the picture album metaphor brought out the following response from an elderly, terminally-ill gentleman : "In one picture I'd be wearing Plus Fours. Those were big bloomer pants." After conveying his love for cars and everything related to cars, he said: "In the picture I see an old Model T Ford." This discussion led him to describe taking car trips with friends, "going down to Minneapolis for Saturday night and coming back."

Dignity Therapy is not about obtaining a complete biography from the patient, nor will every patient feel that his or her history ought to be documented. One elderly gentleman with metastatic lung cancer indicated that drinking alcohol had claimed most of his adult life. There was much that he did not want others to know and large portions of his past that he would just as soon forget. This patient had no desire, even with the help of a therapist, to reconstruct and record his life history. Instead, he used his therapy to seek forgiveness from his estranged family and to wish them luck in avoiding all the mistakes that he had made along the way.

For some patients, the question "When did you feel most alive?" is the equivalent of saying, "Show me your favorite photograph(s)." It can elicit very special moments and detail-filled memories. Even if those recollections are disconnected from the chronological vignettes, which typically emerge from a general scanning of the "photo album," the results can be moving and sometimes, even magical.

Within her Dignity Therapy, a remarkable fifty-six-year-old woman included a beautiful memory of a special gift she created for her grandchildren:

To me, play was always important, picnic lunches and adventure, but one winter when the grandkids were getting older I thought just boxed toys may not be enough. They needed adventure! That October the lake froze over early. Usually you get snow in October, and the lake takes a couple of weeks to freeze over, but this time it was the end of October and no snow. I looked across this marsh filled with what some people call bulrushes, some cattails, the ones with the brown heads. Some of them were so big; they were seven feet tall that fall. I thought, "I'm going to make them an adventure in these bulrushes." So I went with kneepads on my knees, and I wore a life jacket, because I didn't totally trust that ice. I went with a sickle and started slicing the rushes level with the ice. They cut like butter, and I made trails through the bulrushes. Then as the nights got colder, I was lucky, still no snow, but the rushes started to freeze higher, and I could no longer cut with a sickle, so I got a sharp-edged shovel.

Now you have to remember I'm an older lady in town. The end of the lake was just four minutes down our back lane, which was so wonderful, but what were those people thinking with me going out every day, for an hour and a half, for a month and a half at least, making trails? By the time I finished I had almost a mile of trails in amongst the bulrushes. There is delicate art in the marsh, with animal tracks, animal homes, the pines and various clearings. Anything that looked exciting, I went around it, and the trails all joined up. There are also clearings in the marshes, and I came upon a big one, one day and thought, "Perfect. I can have a skating rink in my maze now," and I shoveled that out. Then the snow came, and I thought if we got a big snow storm, I would have to keep the trails cleared out or I'd never have it ready for Christmas. One time we had such a big storm I went out in the middle of the night twice to keep my trails open. If I kept up I could just slide along those trails with my scoop shovel and by Christmas it was ready for the kids.

I had hidden presents like hockey sticks and pucks on the trail, and on Christmas week when they came out, I took the grandchildren to the swamp and said, "Well there's your gift!" They looked puzzled and said, "What gift is that?" I said, "Look! There's an entrance, and there's an adventure waiting." The neat thing was I made a stook out of some bulrushes and blocked off the entrance, so that if you stood back and looked at that marsh, you couldn't even see the maze. To my one little grandson, those bulrushes were like high trees. He couldn't see over them. At first he was scared to go in. They found the opening, and after that they took off. Not only did I have fun with my grandkids, after that the older people in town wanted to go walking in there, and other kids came to play. They never realized how much there was out in that marsh. It was so magical, but at the same time, life hands us good and bad things. I was doing that for my grandkids, but I was dealing with my mother's illness. She was going downhill at this point, and I needed to cry out there. I needed to work off some of my frustrations. I didn't realize until later that that maze had many purposes.

Later, when asked when she felt most alive, she responded, "When I found out I was dying." While she had always been a wonderful mother, grandmother, wife, and daughter, she confessed to taking on too much responsibility for the happiness of others. Whenever she failed to protect those she loved from life's inevitable bumps and disappointments, she would feel responsible and guilty. That all started to change when she learned she was dying. At about that time, she started attending bible classes and had a spiritual awakening. "They started to explain to me what was happening and the more I fed my soul the more it became alive."

In ending her Dignity Therapy, she had the following to say:

Mostly I want my family to know that I'm okay with dying and they must move on. That is the big thing. Don't look back. I was in their lives for a reason. My dying wish is that I be remembered by people stopping off by the river near our town. They should take their socks and shoes off, put their feet in the water, and feel what that's like on a hot summer day. How often we pass by that place and don't stop. Have a to-go coffee. It will stay hot till they get to that river, and I say enjoy the moment. How often we let those moments go. There's so much beauty out there, and you can't get to it, because you don't feel like it today, or it's a long drive. But it's so worthwhile.

Be mindful that there are different kinds of stories or types of disclosures that patients will share.

There are essentially three kinds of stories that patients tend to tell: the "good," the "sad," and what we have come to refer to as the "ugly" stories. The good stories are perhaps those that are easiest to hear and that we intuitively think are the stories patients most like to tell. These are stories that essentially recall a life well lived and convey expressions of gratitude for life's many blessings. These often include expressions of thanks to loved ones or describing how specific individuals enriched their lives. Patients often reflect on the joy of their children and grandchildren and special relationships. Often, they convey specific wishes and hopes for those they will soon leave behind. One woman left the following wish for her recently born granddaughter: "I can only wish her much happiness and good health. And that she finds love everywhere she goes." She also extended the following to her daughters, in anticipation of her quickly approaching death:

I hope that my family has a good serving of faith, because I think this is a time when you really need it. We don't always understand why these things happen. I guess maybe we never understand them but it is always, I think, very helpful if you have faith. Then you can deal with just about anything that is dished out at you. And as much as I don't understand it myself, I'm sure that they will come out of it okay, knowing that I've always loved them, and that they love me. I think that's the most important thing. We all have to lose someone at some time or another. But you know you always have the memories and the good times to remember. You can live with that for the rest of your life, because memories are always very special. And I'm sure it will be the same for them. It will be hard at the beginning, but time heals all wounds. And it will work the same for them.

P. was a fifty-three-year-old recently married man with no children. As a result of a head and neck cancer that required a laryngectomy, he was unable to speak. Therefore, he used a laptop computer to type out his responses to Dignity Therapy.

Interviewer: P, could you tell me about your life, particularly the parts you remember most or remember as most important?

P: The most important parts of my life are those times spent with my wife, especially all the wonderful trips we went on together. Our relationship grew slowly over time, and in fact that's one of my "theories." People, as they spend time together, especially married people, either grow together or grow apart. T and I grew closer over time until we became so very comfortable with each other, in addition to our deep love for each other.

Interviewer: Are there wishes or hopes you have for T.?

P: I wish for T not too long a period where she feels the pain of my loss and that this transforms into more fond memories than a painful sadness. Like how she feels about her parents now. Whenever we would talk of them, in recent years, it would be with a wistful smile and recollection of good times. That's what I hope will come sooner. Also, a happy and contented retirement filled with lots of friends and family to keep her busy. And a puppy.

Other patients will use Dignity Therapy to tell "sad" stories. These are stories that may recall personal tragedy, injustice, or simply recount regrets or previous failures. Although, intuitively, we might consider that telling this kind of story is counter-therapeutic, patients often feel the need to "set the record straight" toward the end of life by offering an explanation for their shortcomings, seeking forgiveness, or in some instances, simply unburdening themselves. One woman with end-stage colorectal cancer felt her care had been mishandled. She recounted "bad, unprofessional behavior" and feeling she had been treated poorly and had not been afforded basic human respect. In recounting her difficult story, she wanted to warn others that "this is possible" and they had best be wary.

Another gentleman with metastatic lung cancer used his Dignity Therapy as an opportunity to recall the shock of learning, at the age of eleven, that he had been adopted. In the course of his session, he explained how this revelation had set the stage for a life of self-loathing, substance abuse, and difficulty maintaining social connections:

From that point on, my self-esteem was at a very, very low end. I didn't feel as though I belonged anywhere, and I felt ashamed. I didn't want anybody to know me. I felt less than desirable and like a ghost in my own home.

Few stories are purely "good" or "sad." This gentleman's generativity document certainly contained elements of both. As a result of meeting his wife and joining Alcoholics Anonymous, he maintained sobriety for thirty years and took responsibility for his personal failures, as well as his successes. In telling his story and rising above his earlier challenges, he was able to place his current illness within a broader context:

I have had a lot of hurt, a lot of anguish, a lot of agony, a lot of confusion, so I have tapped into a source of power which is a little beyond this veil of tears. I am sure that there is something beyond this lifetime. I am sure there is something more. As a matter of fact, I believe that consciousness goes on from here. Now what the big plan is, nobody has ever got back to me on that, but I am sure it is wonderful.

It may be tempting for the therapist to dissuade patients from telling their "sad'" stories. For example, one elderly gentleman with advanced lung cancer began his interview by stating, "Well, I worked up North for about twenty years; that's where I learned to drink." With such an opening, the therapist might be tempted to direct the patient toward more benign or "happier" material. In fact, in this instance—given that this was early in our experience with Dignity Therapy—such maneuvers were attempted. The patient's response, however, indicated that he was not interested in an agenda of trying to "pretty up" his past. His responses lacked poignancy, and the interview quickly stalled. "I don't remember very much about those things . . . but here is what I need to say." At that point he proceeded to speak to his primary objective in undertaking Dignity Therapy; although he felt it was too late to seek forgiveness, he wanted his grandchildren to know who he was, so that they might make better choices than he had.

> Know how to manage and respond to "ugly" stories.

Perhaps the most difficult stories therapists will confront are the so-called ugly stories. These stories are labeled as such because they have the potential to harm the recipient(s) of the generativity document. One woman, for example, described a longstanding, deeply conflicted relationship with her son. Despite her rapidly approaching death, they had not managed to resolve many of the issues that had long maintained the distance between them. At one point, in describing her hopes for her son, she stated, "He's a bum and a free-loader." Clearly, the harshness of these words might be difficult for any child to hear; however, when they reside within a generativity document, forever attesting to disappointment and unresolved conflict, the psychological consequences could be devastating.

We believe that the Dignity Therapist has a responsibility to manage these "ugly" stories and a duty to care, for the patient as well as the recipient(s) of such a document. Perhaps it is helpful to consider the extent to which, under normal clinical circumstances, a care provider might be willing to convey, or participate in conveying, information on the patient's behalf. Should one's willingness to convey information be disconnected from the content of the information itself? Is there a difference in helping patients extend messages of love toward their children, as opposed to articulating messages of disappointment, or perhaps even a sense of loathing directed at specific individuals? While the former seems entirely wholesome and reasonable, the latter should give clinicians pause and solid grounds to remove themselves from the role of willing messenger.

This is not to say that patients are not at liberty to broach whatever issues they like with friends and family; however, they should be encouraged to do so in the *here and now*, rather than from beyond the grave, so to speak. Unlike a real-time conversation, the generativity document does not allow for a dialogue between the patient and recipient, nor is it possible, after the fact, to work through the issues. In the here and now, even difficult conversations can sometimes be healing and cathartic or promote resolution. However, stated within a generatively document, words can amount to a permanent accusation, reprimand, or assault, against which there is no possible defense or retort. Hence, we feel it is the role of the Dignity Therapist to remind the patient that their words are being recorded and could, once delivered have a lasting impact. In response to the dying angry mother, estranged from her son, the therapist might choose to state something like, "If these were the last words you could extend to your son, are they the ones you would want to leave him with, or might there be others you would want him to remember you by?" In this instance, this mother who had initially berated her son and accused him of being a bum, cried and said she would want to tell him how much she loves him, how she wishes she could hold him and then, laughing, added, "and that he ought to get a job!"

Sometimes "ugly" stories are more subtle. As patients become comfortable with speaking, they may actually forget that their words are being recorded and that what they say, the editing process not withstanding, will be read and have an impact on those they choose to share the document with. For example, one jocular gentleman began describing his thoughts about his wife by telling a "dumb blond" joke. The appropriate role of the therapist in this situation was to ask if he really wished this to be part of the generativity document. Mercifully, he did not!

The Dignity Therapist must always be mindful of content that might cause significant harm. There will always be a certain element of judgment in determining the appropriate threshold for intervention. But, if in doubt, it is easy to check with the patient. "You are raising some pretty difficult issues about your [family member] . . . how do you think they will feel hearing this? Have you ever discussed this with them before? Is this something you would consider talking about with them face to face?" It is important that this kind of enquiry take place in the moment, as the opportunity to clarify the appropriate course of action, given the tenuous state of health of many participants, may not recur.

Help patients provide clarity about the details of their stories.

Patients often make assumptions in telling their stories, without explicitly offering the necessary detail for clarity. This can leave their words relatively inaccessible, except for those with sufficient background information. The therapist needs to take an active role in obtaining enough detail, so that the generativity document reads well for loved ones who may later take comfort from it. Remember, the patient may not have the mental wherewithal or energy to think of small details that would otherwise seem second nature. Therefore, the therapist must take on the role of monitoring these issues, so as to ensure that these details are elicited. For example, one elderly gentleman was reflecting on the close and warm relationships that he and his family shared. Although he felt that he had taken the time during the course of his life to share this sense of closeness with his loved ones, nevertheless, he did want to share specific wishes and hopes for his children and particularly his grandchildren. He began referring to them as "my son's eldest boy" and "my daughter's youngest." His closest family members might have been able to sort through who was being identified, but simply having him specify by name who he was talking about, clarified the matter. Later, the names were woven easily into the manuscript, providing his family with a clearer and more accessible record of their father's and grandfather's final written words. Being identified by name, rather than by the less descriptive third person reference the patient had initially used, also provides a sense of having received a benediction of sorts.

Time sequencing is another common clarification issue. Patients might begin telling a story without placing it in a chronological context. Simple questions like, "How old were you at this time?" can provide the necessary clarity and make it easier for the therapist to follow the story and, in turn, know how to direct the patient, should the story start to falter. For example, a middle-aged gentleman with end-stage lung cancer and only a few weeks to live told a complex story of his military experience. His life was a series of adventures, marked by many different moves to various exotic locations around the world. In telling this story, however, he failed to give dates regarding when events took place or his age at any given time. Asking for these details not only provided clarity, but also guided the therapist to the next logical sequence of his history. His last posting, for example, was on Canada's east coast. Knowing this segued logically to an enquiry about how he ended up in the city where he was now hospitalized. This, in turn, led to some important connections about how he was coping with being ill, and his return to a place where he felt he would get good care and family support.

Probably the most common clarity issue encountered in Dignity Therapy is a simple lack of detail. Again, recall that patients are ill, and no matter how well intended they may be, they may lack energy to invest in creating a cogent document that will tell their story or speak on their behalf once they are no longer able to do so. This again is where the skill of the therapist is critical. One particularly ill woman who, as it turned out, was within days of death, simply stated that she loved her daughter and that there was "little else to say." Although this message was straightforward, it was obviously cryptic. In an instance like this, the therapist must try to place himself or herself in the position of the patient and ask, "If I was to tell the story of my child, or to decide on a final message to impart to my child, where would I begin? What issues would I want to cover and what are the things I would not want left unsaid?" Bearing that in mind, the therapist asked the patient to tell him something about her daughter. Although this yielded a few details, like her daughters name, age, and where she was currently attending school, she quickly summarized by saying "how proud" she felt of her daughter. "What do you feel most proud of?" asked the therapist. Again, the patient's answer was general, speaking of how "smart and capable" her daughter had always been. At this point, the therapist invited the patient to provide a much more detailed picture of what exactly she meant: "When you think about you daughter and your feelings of pride, tell me about one or two pictures that come to mind." In this instance, the patient spontaneously recalled her daughter at the age of four, "standing in front of her class pageant . . . in a little green and yellow dress." By encouraging patients to provide this level of detail, they will often come up with additional, meaningful material. In this instance, the patient spoke about how intelligent her daughter had always been, learning to read when she was three, taking piano lessons and playing for her parents and grandparents, and her wish to protect her daughter from a world that all too quickly would become competitive—a world where jealousies can taint relationships. She concluded by saying she was glad to have made the parenting decisions she had made along the way, in that her daughter had turned into such a remarkable young woman.

It is easy for patients to hide behind generalities, not because that is their intent, but because it takes less thought and energy to be vague, than to provide the specifics that would bring their words or recollections to life. Mrs. L. had been a successful businesswoman who came from very humble beginnings. She described how little money she and her family had had as she struggled to learn about the garment industry. In her therapy, she described the first time that she was able to afford to purchase a dress that she helped make at the factory. The therapist, sensing that this was a very meaningful event, asked her to describe the dress. With tears in her eyes, she recalled it being "paisley, and it had a little collar. It had full sleeves, with shades of brown and green, a fake suede belt, and a little bow in the front." She went on to say how she wore that dress "with pride because I paid for it, and because I was part of making it. From then on, I wore everything with pride that I made in the factory." This feeling of accomplishment and self-sufficiency was a fundamental component of this patient's history and personal identity. In response to a question seeking out detail about one seemingly minor event, she was able to share feelings of pride, feelings that defined her sense of self and provided the foundation of her strength, sustaining her over the course of a life long enough to be marked by joy and loss.

Follow the patient's affect as a way of identifying areas to be included in Dignity Therapy.

In attempting to enhance clarity, the therapist risks the interview becoming stilted and bogged down in too much detail. Along the way, clinical judgment and experience will need to guide the therapist in choosing when to seek further information about particular thoughts or events, and when to move on. As a general rule of thumb, following the affect and emotional energy of the interview will serve the therapist well in making these moment-to-moment decisions. For example, one elderly woman was asked to describe her childhood as an attempt to get the interview started. While she offered a few details about where she was born, it was clear that she did so without any particular enthusiasm or energy. Again, Dignity Therapy is not necessarily about biography and not every patient, as this woman illustrates, needs or wants to talk about life history. For her, talking about regrets and the mistakes she had made was the only time in the interview that she spoke with genuine feeling and emotional intensity. Following the affect, in this instance, meant forgoing the recounting of her life story and allowing her to use the document to offer her end-of-life apology to those she felt she had let down and disappointed.

Sometimes the decisions about where to pursue further detail will be less obvious, and the therapist will need to trust his or her own intuition. For example, one gentleman was recalling his early teenage years, giving broad descriptions of where he grew up, attended school, and the makeup of his social network. He then began describing how he passed his summer vacations but, again, in fairly general terms. Following the emotional energy in the session, the therapist asked if he could remember and describe a particular summer scene. The patient lovingly recalled, "getting out in the country on a bike with a pole for fishing, a few miles from the house. In those days, lads didn't take a six pack, but a five pack of Woodbines cigarettes; it was really daring." His obvious pleasure in retelling this episode led to him recounting another summer's tale: "I used to enjoy swimming a lot with the school, and it wasn't too great a distance from the house. We had a spanking new swimming pool close to the house. I can picture it now; I can hear all the screams and shouts. We would have a dip and then go home and have a good Sunday breakfast." The recollection of these halcyon summer days segued into memories of boarding school, and later enrolling in the army.

> Establish critical momentum in the interview and maximize disclosure with minimal expenditure of energy.

Following the emotional energy or affect, using the photo-album metaphor or otherwise eliciting details also helps build momentum within the interview. Without momentum, the interview will feel plodding and difficult for both patient and therapist. The patient will sense that each individual thought must be retrieved independent of the previously shared thought, making the task of creating the narrative burdensome and, in some instances, simply not feasible. The therapist will also have to work extremely hard, helping the patient reach for each consecutive content area to be explored. For example, a critically ill elderly gentleman appeared to have very little energy to invest in his therapy, although he indicated a wish to try. Lack of energy, profound fatigue, and some minor degree of intermittent forgetfulness made the task difficult, although certainly not impossible, to complete. For parts of the interview, the therapist had to structure each question to elicit what, in each instance, was a rather brief, circumscribed answer.

"Where did you grow up?"
"On the farm."
"What do you recall of the farm?"
"A few horses and cows."
"And what kinds of things did you use the horses for?"
"For everything on the farm, plowing and cultivating, whatever."

Given these curt responses, it was obvious the patient felt little enthusiasm in conveying this information, so the task of obtaining it was cumbersome and labored. As it turned out, childhood recollections were not on his mind in undertaking therapy. He was, however, able to speak quite readily about his marital problems, subsequent divorce, and the unraveling of his previously happy life. He felt the document might provide an outlet for an apology to his ex-wife for his various missteps and an explanation of sorts to their two, now adult, children. Tapping into this meaningful area of discourse established a degree of momentum that allowed the therapist to simply sit back, listen, and provide a nonjudgmental, safe space for the story to be told.

> Strike the appropriate therapeutic balance between providing open-ended questioning and imposing more structure.

As a general rule, the more disorganized or fatigued the patient, the more structured the therapy needs to be. Reducing the interview to a series of short questions and answers is the ultimate degree of structure, and should only be imposed when required. While it is conceivable to do therapy in this fashion, this degree of structure may be indicative of a patient who is either too ambivalent or simply too ill to partake in Dignity Therapy. The ideal flow of an interview is one in which the patient is asked a question broad enough to generate an engaged and energized response. If the issues are salient to the patient, the interview will usually proceed easily; if the issues or questions are not meaningful to the patient, the interview will often crawl along or simply come to a complete halt. One sixty-year-old gentleman dying of metastatic lung cancer was reticent to talk about various aspects of his life and the therapist began to feel like he was treading along a series of dead ends. However, when the topic of his childhood was broached, the patient became highly engaged, describing how a chaotic home life had profoundly shaped his core identity and resulted in chronic instability. He spoke about these formative years at length, providing extensive spontaneous detail and doing so with intense feeling. Upon completion, the therapist stated, "You have told me so much about your early years, but haven't said much about the last thirty years. In looking over these past thirty years, are there particular episodes or moments that you feel the need to speak about?" To this, the patient responded, "Not really." Cleary, the appropriate therapeutic maneuver was not to attempt to solicit further biographical information but rather to move into other areas of enquiry, wherein the patient might again become engaged.

Another way of achieving critical momentum is to start broad and then narrow in on detail. Broad questions are those that give the patient the widest range of possible responses. Examples include, Tell me about the parts of your life that you would say are most memorable. What achievements do you feel most proud of? What lessons have you learned from life that you would want to pass along to your loved ones? Notice that the patient has free rein as to where to take the responses. Depending on the patient's energy level and degree of engagement in the process, these broad questions may require little additional prompting to lead to a meaningful generativity document. However, in most instances, patients will require some prompting as their concentration or energy wanes. When this happens, the therapist should then follow up with "detail" questions. Rather than simply asking questions that are likely to evoke very specific answers (Were you happy? Did you have fun? Was it fulfilling?), follow-up questions should invite patients to provide specifics that support their broad question responses. In some instances, the picture-album metaphor may prove helpful. "Imagine that you and I are looking at a photo album of your life. Tell me, in as much detail as you can, about some of the pictures we might see." This picture-album metaphor can also be modified, depending on the direction and flow of the interview. For example, a highly successful businessman was discussing how proud he felt of his children, over and above his various business accomplishments. When asked what it was about his children that made him feel proud, his answers were short and lacking detail. "They are such wonderful people, and have turned out so well." Then the therapist asked the following question: "If we were to look through a photo album of you and your children, could you describe the one or two pictures of your children you would absolutely want me to see?" The patient described a time when he took his daughter to hospital after she broke her arm, and the loving care he and his wife had given in trying to make her comfortable afterward. He also recalled a particular outing of golf with his son and the enjoyment they had shared on that occasion.

Sometimes, simply asking for more detail is all that is required. However, it is best to do so with questions that are open ended, rather then questions that are more likely to elicit brief or circumscribed responses. One elderly gentleman indicated how important his career as a "newspaperman" had been. In speaking about this, however, he reflected on how poorly the papers of today manage their operations compared to in his day. Rather than keeping this conversation general and remote, the therapist invited the patient to personalize his responses with the following questions. "When you look back over your career as a newspaperman, are there particular moments or pivotal milestones or accomplishments that you remember?" The question is broad but asks the patient to share the detailed information that supports the general disclosure of the importance of his career. In his fascinating response, the patient recalled covering the headline story of the "Super Bomb" at Hiroshima, scooping the competing newspaper which, caught off guard, "ran the story on page 34!" Moved by the momentum and poignancy of these memories, he went on to recall other defining moments of his long and illustrious career.

I have had dinner in the White House with President Johnston. How many people get that? It was a lot of fun, and the most interesting thing about it was the crockery. Every president has his own set of dishes. I found that and the marine band the most interesting parts. Then I went over to London, to a Garden Party at Buckingham Palace. Then I went to Rome and met Pope John, the 23rd. My job gave me all these opportunities. Whenever I went to Ottawa, John Diefenbaker would phone up and say, come around to breakfast. He was a strange man and wonderful storyteller. I had dinner once with Trudeau; an unapproachable man, but a brilliant man. I always remember when he was chosen leader of the Liberal Party. I was sitting right below him. When the vote was announced, I don't know whether somebody turned on some lights or what, but his eyes flashed as if he had two flashlight bulbs in them. I always remember that. I remember, too, another of the candidates for the leadership, who was in the passageway under the dais. I went past him, and he was practicing his acceptance speech. He didn't get to read it. So, as I say, it's been a great life."

Understand that some stories may be too painful to tell; give patients permission to withhold recollections that may cause them to feel too vulnerable.

Sometimes following the affect or emotional energy in the therapy will lead to issues or memories that the patient finds too sad or difficult to tell. Conflict, tragedy, ambivalence—all may characterize pivotal events in a patient's life—and yet present too daunting a task for the patient to address, thus rendering them silent. Some forms of psychotherapy may try to guide patients through their conflicted feelings or offer interpretations to address this seeming resistance; Dignity Therapy does neither. The therapist must be respectful of the patient's healthy defenses, even when doing so precludes dealing with specific, underlying issues. One elderly patient described the close relationship she had had with her late husband. "My husband was a gentleman. He was a very, very kind person. And his daughter adored him. If he would have died before her, she would have died. That's how they adored each other. Unfortunately, she died before him . . . but, I don't want to talk about that." At that point, the therapist appropriately replied, "I want you to feel free to talk about the things you want to talk about, and not talk about things you'd rather leave unsaid." As it happened, later in the interview the patient pointed out a picture of her daughter at her bedside and stated, "There are certain pictures I don't mind focusing on about her. Like that picture there with me, in happy times." She went on to describe her daughter's university graduation and receiving that particular graduation picture from her, together with a rose, as a gift. "She was such a wonderful, wonderful person. Some people don't appreciate their children, but I appreciated each and every one of these little things she did for me." Although she did not choose to deal directly with the circumstances surrounding her daughter's death, she was able to include various tender anecdotes and articulate unwavering feelings of love toward her, as she, herself, prepared for death.

Remind the patient that the "time is now."

It is difficult for any of us to imagine our nonexistence. Patients, even those close to death, frequently overestimate the amount of time they have remaining. It is almost as if the expectation of another tomorrow is part of the human condition, one that remains intact, even as tomorrows quickly run out. This can result in patients seemingly deferring to say things, in anticipation of there being other opportunities to do so. Sylvia was a twenty-one-year-old young woman with end-stage leukemia. Diagnosed in her late teens, she had received aggressive therapy, including bone marrow transplantation but, sadly, had now relapsed. She was dependent on transfusions and was quickly running out of curative options. During the course of her Dignity Therapy, she expressed regret for all the things she would probably never have a chance to do or say. In response, the therapist said, "If this was your last chance to say all the things that need saying, what would you say and to whom?" In other words, this served as a gentle way of saying "the time is now." The patient responded by telling her brother that he should not rush into marriage, especially if his motivation for doing so was the possibility of her not living long enough to attend. She also suggested that her family learn to get along and not hold grudges against one another. She told her sister that she should learn to be more confident in her own decisions and judgments, given that after Sylvia's death, she would be likely to take over her role as the family mediator. Dignity Therapy offers patients the chance to say the things they would prefer not be left unsaid. Reminding them of this, in a gentle, nonabrasive manner, allows patients to take full advantage of this opportunity.

As in all aspects of Dignity Therapy, the most important factors determining the

> Pace the therapy to best match the patient's needs and abilities.

number and duration of sessions will be the patient's general state of health, energy, and cognitive capacity. As patients near the end of life, physical energy and mental acuity wax and wane. It is largely up to the therapist to keep track of time and gauge the patient's degree of fatigue and mental ability. Occasionally, patients will surprise you and through their efforts, move beyond initial expectations. One patient seemed to be experiencing difficulty finding a comfortable position due to abdominal discomfort associated with her advanced colorectal cancer. And yet, once the recording started, over the course of nearly one hour, she described her chaotic upbringing, and how "a guardian angel" had taken her under her wing and turned her life around.

Time-keeping is simplified by thinking of the interview as consisting of two primary components. The first component is more biographical and evocative of the life story—more accurately, episodes thereof—elicited by the first questions of the Dignity Therapy question protocol (see also chapter 3):

- Tell me a little about your life history, particularly the parts that you either remember most or think are the most important.
- When did you feel most alive?
- Are there particular things that you would want your family to know about you, and are there particular things you would want them to remember?
- What are the most important roles you have played in your life (e.g., family roles, vocational roles, community service roles)? Why were they so important to you, and what do you think you accomplished within those roles?
- What are your most important accomplishments, and what do you feel most proud of or take most pride in?

Often, within the context of addressing the first question, many facets of the remaining biographical questions, such as what they might want their family to know about them, what roles they considered important, or what accomplishments they take pride in, may already have been addressed. If ever in doubt, the therapist can ask if the patient might have something more to say about a particular issue, topic, or memory. However, early on in the course of the session, usually within the first twenty minutes, the therapist should try to assess whether therapy can be completed in the one session. This decision should be based on the patient's degree of engagement in offering their responses and their clinical status. Should the therapist determine that the patient is up to the task and seems to be providing answers that are rich in content and description, the entire first session may be taken up focusing on biographical material and a more leisurely reconstruction of their story. Another session would then need to be scheduled to focus on the remaining Dignity Therapy questions. The Dignity Therapist, however, must be cautious in taking on this strategy, as patients can deteriorate quickly, which can result in therapy being left incomplete.

Given the dire health of most people who have participated in Dignity Therapy to date, one session is by far the more typical scenario. Hence, be mindful of pacing and the limited time frame, so you can allocate sufficient time to the second and often more emotionally challenging Dignity Therapy questions:

- Are there particular things that you feel need to be said to your loved ones, or things that you would want to take the time to say once again?
- What are your hopes and dreams for your loved ones?
- What have you learned about life that you would want to pass along to others? What advice or words of guidance would you wish to pass along to your [son, daughter, husband, wife, parents, other(s)]?
- Are their important words or perhaps even instructions you would like to offer your family?

These questions are almost invariably emotionally evocative and often elicit replies that are poignant, reflective, and deeply meaningful. One would not want to provide Dignity Therapy without giving the participant an opportunity to respond to these questions in the latter half of the Dignity Therapy protocol. To do this within a one-hour time frame, therapists will need to gauge their time and pace the interview accordingly.

> Before turning off the audio recorder, always provide the patient a chance to get in a final word.

For most patients, one recorded session, occasionally two, is all that is required and realistic. Keep in mind that every Dignity Therapy session requires four or more patient contacts (including the recorded meeting). Aim to have all patient contacts completed in about one week. The first meeting is usually about twenty minutes and is intended to explain the intervention, find out some basic background information (establishing the "frame" of Dignity Therapy), and plan the therapy itself (identify if there are content themes or issues that the patient wants to address).

The second contact is the recorded Dignity Therapy session itself, which usually takes about one hour. Depending on the patient's energy level and degree of engagement, an additional meeting may be scheduled to finish any remaining questions. Before turning off the audio recorder, it is good practice to provide the patient with an opportunity to have a final word. "In creating this permanent record, are there other things that you would like included?" Not infrequently, the idea that this is a final chance to speak their mind, at least at that particular moment, either elicits something new or moves patients to underscore or highlight, for the sake of emphasis, something they may have already said.

By the time the Dignity Therapy session is nearing its end, the therapist should feel that patients have had every opportunity to speak their mind, share their story, and say all that they feel, under the circumstances, is critical to be said. It is really quite extraordinary how much can be covered in a single session. As an aside, when I teach Dignity Therapy, I usually conduct an actual interview, either with a patient or a simulated patient, in the presence of the trainees. At the conclusion of these demonstrations, I often ask, "How many of you feel you know the essence of who this person is?" It is humbling and gratifying to see the room fill with raised hands. A successful session should elicit this kind of response, providing a sense that the essence of this person has been captured by their words, musings, reminiscences, and reflections.

Be sure to leave some time for a debriefing with the patient.

Once the audio recorder has been turned off, take a moment to debrief with the patient. "How was that for you? Are you pleased with how things went? Was that more tiring than you anticipated? I noticed that some parts were quite emotional—was that hard for you?" These are some of the possible questions you might ask, acknowledging that the patient has invested considerable energy into an important process. In most instances, the debriefing will be short and positive. However, should the patient have some misgivings or anxiety about what transpired during the course of the interview, it is better to find that out immediately, rather than having the patient worry about it until the next appointment.

Finally, before leaving the patient, be sure to review the next steps of the Dignity Therapy protocol. Remind him or her that you will have the audio recording transcribed in its entirety and that you will then edit the document. Try to provide a realistic sense of the time frame, bearing in mind that an ethos of rapid turnaround and immediacy also lends credence to their words and to the process they are engaged in. If Dignity Therapy is working well and is appropriately resourced, the editing and the follow-up appointment(s) should take place within the next three to four days. As previously indicated, a shorter turn-around time under more dire circumstances is possible but needs to be planned in advance.

The third meeting takes about twenty minutes. (Recall that the interview must be transcribed and edited between the second and third meetings.) The purpose of the third meeting is to review the edited transcript with the patient. The patient may opt to read the transcript or have you read it aloud in its entirety. Patients usually find this quite moving and very meaningful. It also provides an opportunity to determine whether there are any corrections, additions, or deletions that need to be made. These amendments to the edited transcript should be made as directed by the patient. Keep the audio recorder handy, in case any of the patient's thoughts need to be recorded verbatim for later inclusion in the transcript.

> Toward the end of her Dignity Therapy session, one woman asked her young adult son to forgive her for not having disclosed the identity of his father—her long estranged husband. By the time she considered doing so, it was too late, as he had long since died. She was unable to provide her son any real explanation, other than an irrational fear that knowing his father might somehow have threatened their own relationship.

Occasionally, patients may provide some insights about the manuscript that might help inform the editing process: "I shouldn't have said that." "I may not have said enough about my other daughter." Appropriate changes can be made to the manuscript to reflect the patient's wishes.

In the fourth meeting, the patient is presented with the final generativity document. The protocol for returning this document was informed by one of our first patients taking part in a Dignity Therapy clinical trial. At the conclusion of her interview, she was asked how the document ought to be returned. Her advice was to place it in an attractive but modest blue folder, and have the document itself printed on some better quality paper. While I have seen variation across different sites, our practice is to print the document on bond grade, beige paper, and to place it in a blue, light-weight binder.

It is humbling to be the recipient of a person's life story, to listen to the lessons they have learned, the blessings they wish to convey, and the legacy they wish to leave behind. Dignity Therapists in Canada, the United States, Denmark, England,

Scotland, Portugal, Spain, China, and Australia have all been touched by the opportunity to do this work, invariably using words such as "honor" and "privilege" to describe their experiences. This is no ordinary conversation you have just taken part in, nor ordinary disclosures you have just heard. They represent a lifetime's accumulation of experiences and insights and, if you have done your job right, they have the potential to resonate across generations to come. Be sure to thank the patient for the honor and privilege of sharing those words with you.

REFERENCES

1. Chochinov HM, Hack T, McClement S, Kristjanson L, Harlos M. Dignity in the terminally ill: a developing empirical model. *Soc Sci Med.* 2002;54(3):433–443.
2. Chochinov HM. Dignity-conserving care--a new model for palliative care: helping the patient feel valued. *JAMA.* 2002;287(17):2253–2260.
3. Chochinov HM, Hack T, Hassard T, Kristjanson LJ, McClement S, Harlos M. Dignity therapy: a novel psychotherapeutic intervention for patients near the end of life. *J Clin Oncol.* 2005;23(24):5520–5525.
4. Chochinov HM, Hack T, Hassard T, Kristjanson LJ, McClement S, Harlos M. Dignity and psychotherapeutic considerations in end-of-life care. *J Palliat Care.* 2004;20(3):134–142.

5

THE GENERATIVITY DOCUMENT

Why bother with sick people, why try to save them, if they're not worth acknowledging? When a doctor refuses to acknowledge a patient, he is, in effect abandoning him to his illness.

—Anatole Broyard

Mr. M. was particularly ill when he was referred for Dignity Therapy. His wife, who was caring for him at home with support from community palliative care services, was quite keen for him to be offered the chance to participate in Dignity Therapy. She felt that it might be good for his spirits, and at some level, that it might benefit her and her two daughters. She decided to sit in on the Dignity Therapy interview, both to offer her husband support and to be sure that he covered some of the key issues she hoped he might address. In spite of her best efforts, however, she was concerned that his responses sometimes "wandered" and that she had to guide him more than she had anticipated to elicit some of his important memories and words of comfort for his children. Before reading the final edited manuscript, she confided her anxiety that the interview may not have "captured his essence." However, after reading the edited document, she was "surprised and relieved" that she was able to see—as she knew her children would be able to see—the loving husband, the caring father, the playful personality, and the generous spirit reflected in the final, edited version of his generativity document.

In nearly every country where Dignity Therapy training has taken place, the task of editing the verbatim transcript arouses curiosity and some degree of trepidation.

After all, these transcripts are often the final recorded words of the patient; is it right to edit or change them in any way? What is the rationale for doing so? How does one know if the editing is in keeping with the patient's wishes? Can the requisite skills to edit be readily acquired? Does the requirement to edit reduce the feasibility of doing Dignity Therapy in various palliative and end-of-life care settings? These are very legitimate questions; to feel comfortable with Dignity Therapy, each needs to be frankly and fully addressed.

THE RATIONALE FOR EDITING DIGNITY THERAPY TRANSCRIPTS

Why bother editing Dignity Therapy transcripts considering that, in most instances, these will be the patient's final recorded words? Is it presumptuous or perhaps even wrong to tamper with or in any way change what the patient actually said or, more to the point, how they said it? This is a critical question and one that needs to be settled before proceeding to describe the task of editing a Dignity Therapy transcript.

To begin the discussion, it is helpful to return to the therapeutic contract established with Dignity Therapy participants. The role of the therapist is to enable the patient to accomplish something that could not be done without therapeutic assistance and guidance. Those enrolled in Dignity Therapy are facing life-threatening and life-limiting circumstances. Typically, patients lack the time, energy, and mental ability to accomplish many tasks, let alone one that consists of constructing and organizing a detailed and reflective document. Even without these limitations, many patients might feel intimidated at the prospect of trying to document some of their heartfelt thoughts or feelings, knowing that these words will achieve longevity beyond the measure of their own days. Dignity Therapy provides patients a means of overcoming many of the obstacles that normally prevent them from taking on this type of legacy-generating task. Agreeing to Dignity Therapy includes the patient's willingness to accept the aid of the therapist. In other words, patients consent to participate in a process that will produce a detailed generativity, legacy-preserving document, with the understanding that the therapist will provide the means by which they can succeed.

Lack of mental fortitude may disincline many patients from taking on a legacy-making task, particularly one they anticipate might not "turn out right." Each of us is invested in being heard correctly and in hoping that our words will accurately reflect what we feel. This is especially true when those words are to be written down, read by others, and serve as a permanent indicator of who and what we are or were. Under these circumstances, few patients would want to "get it wrong." No one wants to sound confused, come across disjointedly, or be portrayed in a fashion that is less than coherent. Patients also want their words to be worthy of their thoughts, feelings, and recollections. Ultimately, what patients want to see captured in their generativity document is an accurate reflection of themselves. Toward the end of life, it is difficult to imagine a more precious gift for one to leave behind.

Our therapeutic contract with patients is to safeguard their dignity by ensuring that they are as successful in Dignity Therapy as possible. It is, therefore, our responsibility to help them achieve, not simply what they could achieve on their own, but rather, all they might wish and deserve to achieve. In essence, the Dignity Therapist is saying, "Together, we can do this and we can do this right." This means that disorganized or distracted thinking is not treated as sacrosanct, simply because it happens to be part of the patient's narrative. Instead, we adhere to our therapeutic commitment when we help patients reach beyond their grasp, both during the course of the interview and during the process of editing the manuscript. Polishing a rough edge, compensating for disorganization, eliminating extraneous content that might diminish from the whole are all editorial procedures that, judiciously applied, will yield a final generativity document that the patient could have produced had they been feeling well enough to do so. To settle for anything less is a breach of the Dignity Therapy contract.

TRANSCRIBING THE AUDIO RECORDED INTERVIEW

Before describing the editing process, a few comments on transcribing the audio recorded interview are necessary. The transcript, after all, provides all the raw material available to construct the edited generativity document. Hence, details regarding how it is produced are important.

Beginning with the transcriptionist, several issues are noteworthy. The content of Dignity Therapy is almost always emotionally evocative. Even the most straightforward of stories may take on striking poignancy when told by someone nearing the end of life. Transcripts often contain words of love, regret, anguish, longing, and grief—in essence, the vast panorama of human experience. Transcriptionists require strong and accurate typing skills, but they also require the maturity to take on this special task. In selecting transcriptionists, bear in mind the emotional nature of the recordings. People chosen for this task must be prepared to listen to this type of content and be offered opportunities to share their emotional responses.

Mrs. A., a regular Dignity Therapy transcriptionist, described how upsetting listening to the recordings of young people could be. She recalled being moved to tears on many occasions, having to take occasional breaks from her work before feeling ready to return to the task at hand. She also felt strongly that the job of transcribing patients' final words, unlike any other typing contracts she held, was "profoundly special and meaningful." She approached this task with a sense of "responsibility and privilege" unique to this job. She also expressed a sense of curiosity regarding how the initial raw product she typed would be transformed into a generativity document, and hoped that it would provide the patient comfort.

Fully discuss the purpose and content of Dignity Therapy, the nature of Dignity Therapy recordings, and the very direct and critical role that the transcriptionist plays in the overall process. How prospective transcriptionists respond to this discussion should form part of the evaluation of their suitability for the task. Transcriptionists must also understand the importance of timeliness in this work. Although it is not realistic to expect someone to drop all of their other obligations to transcribe, verbatim, a Dignity Therapy recording, nonetheless, the task must be done quickly. It should be completed in a time frame of one to three days.

Be mindful that time is usually working against us. For that reason, having a cadre of transcriptionists (four to six, depending on the size of the Dignity Therapy program) is ideal. So long as they can collectively provide adequate coverage, the flow and tempo of the Dignity Therapy protocol can proceed unimpeded. As Dignity Therapy services evolve, various models for timely transcription will no doubt emerge to accommodate local contexts and circumstances. Some centers may consider incorporating this task into already existing medical transcription services; where those services are overtaxed, a parallel system of independent contractors may be more attractive. Bearing in mind fiscal considerations, some palliative care programs may explore using competent volunteer transcriptionists, while others might examine the role that voluntary organizations such as local hospices or similar palliative care organizations could play. Depending on the length of the interview, the time required for each individual transcription ranges from two to three hours; verbatim transcription usually takes about two to three times the length of the actual interview to complete. The amount of time required for any one patient is not onerous, and completing the transcription as soon as possible helps deliver the message, "Your words are important, as is the task of having them permanently and carefully documented." Systemic solutions for transcription must include rapid—and thus dignity-conserving or dignity-affirming—turnaround times. Once appropriate transcriptionists have been engaged, stress the following points:

- **Overall approach.** Transcribing a Dignity Therapy interview is a special and important task. Being able to find the needed time and feeling personally invested in the process will make this task not only feasible but, by all reports, emotionally and intellectually gratifying.

- **Timing.** It is critical that the work of Dignity Therapy transcription be completed as soon as possible. This means that in taking on a job, the transcriptionist commits to completing the job within no more than a three-day time frame.

- **Confidentiality.** The Dignity Therapy transcript will contain highly detailed and personal information. The transcriptionist must maintain patient confidentiality and adhere to all locally relevant institutional policies, professional codes, and legislation regulating personal health information.

- **Generativity document layout.** The layout of the transcript can greatly facilitate the editing process and, thus, is a standard element of the Dignity Therapy protocol. Given that the transcript will read like a conversation between the interviewer and the patient, each new exchange of dialogue should be labeled to indicate the current speaker. Because the patient's words are the only words of particular importance, the interviewer can simply be labeled "Interviewer" or, according to their full title the first time it appears, and then abbreviated; for instance, "Dr. Smith," and thereafter "Dr. S." or "Interviewer." The patient's dialogue, on the other hand, should be clearly labeled each time, initially using the full name, and subsequently using the name by which they prefer to be addressed, as indicated during their interview; for instance, Mrs. Rose Johnston and Rose, respectively.

Interviewer: Mrs. Johnston, before we get too far into the interview, can you tell me how you would like me to address you?

Mrs. Rose Johnston: I'm not sure I understand what you mean.

Interviewer: Well, would you like me to call you Mrs. Johnston or would you prefer Rose?

Rose: Oh, I see what you are saying; everyone calls me Rose, so that would suit me just fine.

Interviewer: So Rose, to begin with, why don't you tell me a little bit about yourself and your life, particularly the things that you feel are most important or that you would most want your family to know.

Rose: My, that's not an easy question . . . to be honest, I'm not really quite sure where to begin.

Interviewer: That's perfectly understandable. Why don't I see if I can help you, OK?

- **Equipment.** Transcriptionists need to remember that the patients whose words they will be transcribing are invariably quite sick. The various encumbrances of illness can make it challenging to accurately discern the patient's words. It is not uncommon for the transcriptionist to have to review a segment of dialogue several times, in order to make the transcription accurate.

Good quality transcription equipment is essential. Either analog or digital recording will do, depending on which the therapist is most familiar and which best accommodates the local protocol requirements. For instance, digital recordings can be sent effortlessly and electronically between the Dignity Therapist and the transcriptionist. This must be done over networks that have sufficient security, however, so as not to jeopardize the privacy of anyone involved.

- **Accuracy.** The transcriptionist should be instructed to transcribe the document as accurately as possible. Although a straight forward directive, this is by no means easily achieved. When patients are very ill, it is not unusual for voice volume to wax and wane. Coughing, wheezing, and shortness of breath are but some of the realities of advanced illness, which might further complicate the task of accurate transcription. Transcriptionists should be forewarned of these challenges and take breaks when their concentration is starting to fade. They should also be aware that verbatim accuracy is less of an issue in documenting the words of the interviewer, whose comments will largely be edited or reconstructed. On the other hand, every effort should be made to document the patient's words as accurately as possible. If certain words of phrases are inaudible, [ ] can be used to denote periodic lapses or gaps. Partial documentation of what was said is better than none whatsoever, and may allow the editor/therapist to reconstruct the essence of the patient's intended words. For example:

Interviewer: You were starting to say something about your daughter.

   Lydia: Yes [ ] so beautiful.

Interviewer: And tell me Lydia, when you describe her as beautiful, are you connecting that to a particular memory you might describe for me?

Lydia: Yes [ ] I was thinking about her first day of school and [ ] pretty, new dress she wore.

Clearly, the patient's intent, while not entirely captured by the transcriptionist, was to convey how beautiful she remembers her daughter looking in her pretty new dress on her first day of school. The edited version would be likely to read as follows:

Lydia: "She was so beautiful. I was thinking about her first day of school and the pretty new dress she wore."

Sometimes it is not the illness, but rather being caught up in the emotion of Dignity Therapy that can hamper the clear articulation and subsequent transcription of the patient's words. Generally, we do not ask transcriptionists to record the emotional tone of the interview. However, if either laughter or tears cause a significant disruption in the interview, it can be helpful to have this noted. Often, the editor/therapist will remember these "feelings." Should nonverbal expressions of emotion be quite prominent, it need not be documented in every instance, but rather, selectively—at the transcriptionist's discretion—in order to remind the editor/therapist of the emotional tone. These reminders of tone can help inform the process of editing.

> Interviewer: And what do you recall happening next?
> Frank: [ ] (laughter) [ ] it's hard to describe [ ] Maybe you just had to be there!

In this instance, the inclusion of tone clarifies the intended meaning, whereas the words themselves convey a message that could be interpreted either way.

- **Word processing and program compatibility**. It is important that the transcriptionist use the same word processing program as the editor/therapist uses in the editing process. Whatever program is selected, it is highly recommended that it include a "track changes" function. This has quality assurance implications, in that it enables all Dignity Therapy documents to be viewed in three versions: the original unedited transcript, the tracked changes edited version (that displays all additions and deletions, usually with color coding and margin notations) and the final, edited version. This enables Dignity Therapists to share their work with other therapists, supervisors, or mentors, allowing critical feedback on both their therapeutic strengths and weaknesses and their editing skills.
- **Electronic transcript transfer**. It is vital that the therapist/editor receive an electronic version of the transcription. This allows the editing to be completed, using the "track changes" function of the word processing program. Because of confidentially issues, the transfer of transcripts by e-mail must be done with appropriate caution and security measures (using encryption or other appropriate safeguards); alternatively, it can be saved to and delivered in a CD or USB-memory stick format.
- **Debriefing**. Transcriptionists should be asked about their experience of doing this work on a regular basis. As previously indicated, the content of Dignity Therapy is often emotionally evocative; even emotionally neutral material can resonate in ways that are quite poignant, given the circumstances of the people who partake in Dignity Therapy. Simply listening to the transcriptionist's responses can provide important support and gauge whether the individual is well-suited to this work. On occasion, it can be very helpful—and rather

enlightening—to bring the transcriptionists together to share their experiences and feelings with one another about doing this unique work.

EDITING THE VERBATIM TRANSCRIPT

Once the transcribing is completed and the transcript delivered in an electronic format, the editing can begin in earnest. Like every other facet of Dignity Therapy, a dual sense of immediacy and respect are essential. The message being given with the pacing and tone must be clear and unequivocal: "What you have to say is valuable, and the process of retrieving your words is too important to be delayed." Just because the interview has been completed does not mean that there is any slackening of this approach. This needs to be made explicit to the patient, who should be told at the conclusion of the Dignity Therapy interview that the transcription and editing process will commence immediately, and should take no more than a few days.

The task of editing should be approached with feelings of deference and responsibility. During the course of this task, the words and the legacy of another individual, quite literally, are in the editor's hands. Besides this all-important attitude, editors are well advised to create a comfortable space for doing this particular work. Katherine Cullihall, a senior research nurse and experienced Dignity Therapist at the Manitoba Palliative Care Research Unit, suggests one needs a cup of tea or coffee, a computer and printer, a comfortable chair, and time without distractions.

The ideal Dignity Therapy editor, at least in our experience, is the person who conducted the Dignity Therapy interview. Unlike anyone else who might take on this task, the Dignity Therapist has participated in the interview process and has heard, first hand, everything the patient has said. This provides some privileged insights, conveyed either explicitly or in a more nuanced manner. The therapist may recall words the transcriptionists missed; but more important, he or she will remember the patient's intended message, the things meant to be emphasized; what issues were conveyed with emotional intensity and what material may simply have mattered less. While this has obvious resource implications, as Dignity Therapists improve their skills, editing becomes more efficient and less time consuming. A well-facilitated Dignity Therapy results in an easier task of editing. In the hands of experienced therapists, editing usually takes twice the time required for the interview itself i.e. a one hour interview should take about two hours to edit.

To begin, editors are well advised to set up the font type and size of their word processing package to something they find easy to read (e.g. Garamond 14; with line spacing set at 1.5–2.0; both the left and right margins can be set at 1.5 cm). Then, turn on the tracking function, in order to assist you and others wishing to review changes in the document. This creates excellent quality assurance and education opportunities. When the original transcripts are received, there may be portions missing from the dialogue. On occasion, the editor may have to review the audio tape; having participated in the interview, the therapist is in the best position to understand things that may have been missed by the transcriptionist.

The actual editing process is divided into four primary tasks or stages. While the sequencing of these tasks is not critical, it is essential that they each be carried out. These tasks consist of (1) cleaning up the transcript; (2) clarifying the transcript; (3) correcting time sequences; and (4) finding a suitable ending. As editors gain experience and become more adept, efficiencies will develop, allowing for multiple tasks to be handled simultaneously. Whatever the experience of the editor, it is advisable that quiet time be set aside so that concentration and care can be optimal. Katherine Cullihall describes her approach to editing as follows:

> I want to make sure that each manuscript comes out being unique to that person; this isn't just a cookie-cutter approach. Editors must be sensitive to what they cut or add, always being true to the participant's words and wishes. Editing sometimes feels like putting together a puzzle; you have all the pieces, you just need to fit them together so they tell the patient's story in the best way possible. Doing this work is a privilege; you are given someone's words, words they may not have shared with anyone else and are being trusted to make sure that their voice and their message will be heard by the people they love and care about most.

Cleaning Up the Transcript

Spoken language is different from written language. The first task of editing is to clean up the manuscript so that it reads more like prose than like a recorded conversation. For example, Brenda was a forty-two-year-old woman with advanced, end-stage cancer. She and her husband had divorced a number of years earlier, resulting in Brenda raising her daughter, Amanda, on her own. Near the beginning of the interview, Brenda was asked to reflect on the parts of her life that she felt were most important.

> Brenda: Well, I do have some memories of my mom, but there are just a few. So I think, uh, parts that I remember my mom. As things important in my life; making really good friends. Lots of really good friends. Working, you know that was important to me. Up until Amanda came along that was far more important but yes. . . . I did enjoy my work and traveling and seeing different things, and I wish I could be that I was still in that field.

Notice that typical of spoken language, there are thoughts and sentences that are incomplete and add little if anything by way of clarity. There are also occasional non-starters and filler words (e.g. "you know"). All of these hallmarks of spoken language are easily addressed in the initial task of editing. After editing, the previous passage reads as follows:

> I do have some memories of my mom, but just a few. As for things important in my life: making really good friends, lots of really good friends. Working was important to me. Up until Amanda came along, that was far more important. I did enjoy my work and traveling and seeing different things. I wish I could still be in that field.

Notice how much better this reads. In the order that changes were made, the word "well" has been deleted, as it suits spoken language and less so written prose. The sentence "So I think, uh, parts that I remember my mom" can be deleted, without losing her thought about her memories of her mother. Eliminating the words "you know" converts the sentence "Working, you know, that was important to me" to "Working was important to me." The phrase "but yes" has been deleted from the beginning of the sentence "but yes . . . I did enjoy my work," without changing the meaning of the phrase. Finally, the last sentence, which originally contained the phrase "*and I wish I could be that I was still in that field*" has been reworked into two sentences and the syntax changed so that it becomes, "I wish I could still be in that field."

This notion of cleaning up is particularly easy to apply to the voice of the interviewer. As much as possible, the interviewer's words should be cleaned up and, where possible, eliminated. This helps reduce the likelihood that the transcript will read like a conversation rather than prose. Hence, the rule of thumb is that the interviewer's words should remain only to the extent that they provide clarity. For example, at one point in the interview, Brenda describes her daughter, Amanda, as follows: "Amanda is delightful and smart and funny *and generous. I always see wonderful qualities in her and they seem to come to her so naturally.*" At that point Brenda needed some prompting, leading the interviewer to ask, "Do you have a picture in your mind as you talk about those qualities of Amanda? Is there a time that you are thinking of?" This helped Brenda recall the way Amanda was in school, how easily she made friends and how people spoke of her. In the final edited manuscript, the interviewer's words were eliminated, leaving the following uninterrupted paragraph:

> Amanda is delightful and smart and funny and generous. I always see wonderful qualities in her and they seem to come to her so naturally. Amanda makes friends

easily, and blends in easily with her environment and people. She is really, just likeable. "Amanda, Amanda, Amanda" is what you hear in the class or at school.

Anything in the transcript can be edited—resulting in the subtlest to the most substantive of changes. Certainly, words that patients might later deem embarrassing, words they regret saying, anything that could be damaging to surviving loved ones, all of these can readily and easily be dealt with in the editing process.

One elderly gentleman living in a hospice felt that he might have made too many disclosures in his therapy. Specifically, he worried that his sons might feel hurt in hearing about his feelings toward his ex-wife and the less than perfect job he had done as a father following his divorce. In reviewing the transcript with him, it appeared that he had been quite sensitive in addressing these issues and this impression was shared with him. As a result, he felt more comfortable and reassured. He was advised to review the transcript and, of course, was reassured that the document could be further edited and that the ultimate decision regarding its disposition would be his.

Clarifying the Transcript

At times, patients may say something that they perceive to be quite obvious but that later reads less than clear. Even the initial changes that are made with cleaning up may not clarify these instances of ambiguity. For example, early on in Brenda's therapy, the interviewer asked her why she was participating. According to the original transcript, her answer read, "doing this for Amanda so she has a bit of me to know." With some minor clarification, the statement is reworked to read as follows: "I am doing this for Amanda, so she has a bit of me to know." Notice that the original voice of the patient is entirely preserved, and even though some words have been added to the transcript [I am], they are in keeping with the patient's tone and "voice." Adding the words, "I am . . . doing this for Amanda" is quite different than changing the words to, "My reasons for participating in this legacy exercise for Amanda . . ." This, of course, would have been far too formal and out of tune with the patient's speaking style.

Sometimes, clarification will take slightly more work, in that it may require that one phrase be incorporated with another. For example, Frank was a sixty-two-year-old gentleman with an aggressive head and neck cancer, whose death was quickly approaching. He identified his wife and two children as being most important in his life, with the original transcript reading as follows:

Interviewer: And the first question I want to ask you is, what do you remember as being important in your life, or times that you remember as being important and why?

Frank: Well, getting married for one.

Interviewer: Yes.

Frank: And having my children.

Interviewer: Yes.

Frank: And uh, well that's life. Those are the two important things in my life.

Interviewer: Yeah. Can you tell me about getting married? Can you tell me when you and your wife met?

Frank: We met when we were both sixteen years old.

Interviewer: Sixteen . . . and your wife's first name? Just for the record . . .

Frank: Heather.

Interviewer: Heather, yeah. You were sixteen.

With the editorial changes, the prior passage reads as follows:

Interviewer: Frank, can you tell me about your life, particularly the parts you remember the most or remember as being most important?

Frank: Well, getting married for one, and having my children. And well, that's life. Those are the two important things in my life. Heather, my wife, and I met when we were both sixteen years old.

Notice, to provide clarity, the editor combined the sentences, "Well, getting married for one" and, "And having my children." Furthermore, the patient's wife's name, Heather, was inserted into the sentence, "We met when we were both sixteen years old," resulting in the edited version, "Heather, my wife, and I met when we were both sixteen years old."

At times a single word or phrase from a prior sentence may need to be transplanted. In other instances, entire sentences or paragraphs may need to be moved, should doing so add clarity or chronological coherence. For example, later in the interview, Frank indicated that his early years—prior to age sixteen—had been horrible, and not a time in his life he wanted to speak about. In essence, this man was saying that life began at sixteen, when he met and fell in love with his wife, Heather.

Later in the interview with Frank, the following brief exchange took place:

Interviewer: And I'm just going to backtrack a little bit, if . . . and see if you want to go there or not. Um, you talked about the time when you were sixteen that you met Heather. What was your life like before you were sixteen? Did you want to talk about important things during that time?

Frank: Uh, before sixteen?

Interviewer: Uh hmm.

Frank: Well, there's not much that I want to talk about.

Interviewer: OK, that's fine. I just wanted to check it out because that . . . that's fine. No problem. So sixteen is when life started to . . .

Frank: Yeah.

Interviewer: be good for you?

Frank: Up til then, well . . .

Interviewer: Yeah.

Frank: It wasn't good.

Interviewer: OK. We'll leave that part.

From this segment of the transcript, the following sentence could be constructed and inferred: "Up until then, life wasn't good." This could then be appended to the prior piece of dialogue, referring to when he met his wife at age sixteen, with the final result looking like this: "Well, getting married for one, and having my children. And well, that's life. Those are the two important things in my life. Heather, my wife, and I met when we were both sixteen years old. Up until then, life wasn't good."

Often, when there is more than one interview, the follow-up session(s) will provide material that can be placed within the context of the first transcript. On occasion, people may just pick up where they left off in the prior session, but more often, they will provide elaboration to material previously shared. For example, one woman, who had said a great deal about her daughter during the first interview, did not feel she had shared sufficient material about her son. The second session, therefore, focused largely on anecdotes she recalled about his life. This material was later seamlessly combined with the first transcript, where it best fit chronologically.

Correcting Time Sequences

Patients do not necessarily talk about things in the sequence that they occurred, but rather in the order that they happen to recall them. This is no problem whatsoever. In fact, spontaneous recollection is often accompanied by optimal energy and engagement. On the other hand, reading a generativity document that is not chronologically coherent can be problematic. Time dissequences can make the document less accessible and difficult to follow. In other words, the order in which things are disclosed and the optimal order in which they appear in the generativity document are not necessarily the same.

Once the editing process has cleaned up and clarified the transcript, correcting time sequences is relatively easy. This is often as simple as moving anything from a sentence to entire paragraphs elsewhere within the document. Doing so in a fashion that follows the chronological thread of the patient's story will make for a much more coherent and readable document; this also underscores the importance of clarifying details regarding time and the sequence of events during the Dignity Therapy session itself.

As in all aspects of editing, the guiding principle in addressing time sequences should be whether it adds to the clarity and overall quality of the document. For instance, on one occasion, an elderly woman was discussing her feelings toward her middle-age son. In the process of doing so, she shared her impression that he embodied many of the fine qualities of her late and much loved father. Both, in her opinion, were men with a unique creative flare and gentle disposition. While this was a lovely comparison and fit well with her remarks about her son, the mention of her father evoked vivid memories of her early childhood and the fashion in which her parents had markedly influenced her own world view. These aspects of the transcript were easily moved earlier into the document, thereby providing a rich context for later life events she had already shared, including her time in the workforce, meeting her husband, and later starting a family.

Finding a Suitable Ending

Part of the editor's task is to determine what would make a suitable ending for the Dignity Therapy document. In most instances, when patients are coming to the end of their session, the conversation may turn to rather routine issues, such as feeling fatigued, needing some aspect of care attended to, or feeling it is time to turn off the recorder. Be mindful that patients sometimes say things that are quite poignant and lovely when they know the opportunity to record their words is coming to a close. For the most part, things that happen to be said toward the end of the session are strikingly anticlimactic, compared with the often profound, poignant, or emotional issues that have been raised during the course of the interview. Just because the final thing someone happened to say at the end of their session was that they needed a bathroom in no way commits the Dignity Therapy editor to use this as the closing statement of the manuscript. Given the importance of this document, to do so would be an affront to the process of Dignity Therapy and certainly not in keeping with the therapeutic commitment to make this document the very best that it can be.

With that in mind, during editing, it is important to watch for a statement that might make an appropriate ending. For instance, at some point the patient may have said, "I don't know whether I always made every right decision, but my friends and family know I did my best." Perhaps in an earlier response ,the patient might have said something reflective and summative: "It's been a good life" or "Once you've told the people you love that you love them, there isn't much left to say." These statements, composites of actual endings from Dignity Therapy transcripts, strike a tone that is respectful to the process, in sync with the overall tone of the document, and aesthetically, a fitting way to end a generativity document.

The Patient Has the Final Say

Once the manuscript has been shaped and polished to the best of the therapist/editor's ability, it is returned to the patient for final approval. This critical element of editing requires the Dignity Therapist to read the entire edited manuscript to the patient, allowing for any final corrections to be made. (Alternatively, should they prefer, patients may choose to read the manuscript themselves.) In many instances, this is a profound experience for the patient. Hearing a summary of their reminiscences, thoughts, feelings, and wishes can be deeply moving for patients and is usually very gratifying. I recall one gentleman who was moved to tears, as he recognized himself in a document he so worried might not capture the essence of who he was and all that he wanted to say. Changes can be small, that is, the correction of a name, date, or location. Sometimes, because not everything will be caught at the interview, individual words or names of people or places can be checked with the patient during the read-through. In other instances, changes can be large. For example, the woman who realized how little she had said about her son needed to correct this oversight by adding additional content in order to feel satisfied with her Dignity Therapy document. This process allays anxiety on both sides of the patient-therapist equation. The therapist can be assured that the editing is accurate and true to the patient's words. The patient, on the other hand, can listen to the edited version of the transcript and ensure that it is satisfactory. In essence—and as it should be—the patient gets the final say.

Chapter 6 will provide two complete unedited transcripts and their edited counterparts. However, the transcript below provides a very short example of Dignity Therapy, making it easier to see where the editing decisions were made. The patient in this instance was a seventy-one-year-old gentleman who was very close to death. Although because of illness his Dignity Therapy was atypically brief, his wife and four children were nevertheless very pleased with the final result.

> Interviewer: George, I am wondering if you could tell me a little bit about your life, or perhaps share with me some of the things that you felt were especially important.
>
> George: The purchase of my new cars over the years has always been an exciting thing for me and so those are in my mind more important things.
>
> Interviewer: Do you know what made those important for you? Do you remember what made them important, the cars?

George: I don't really know, I just know that they were an exciting thing to get involved in. They make me feel good. You know, generally speaking, they just gave me a good feeling.

Interviewer: Do you remember one in particular?

George: Well, I guess probably the '49 Mercury. That is still a very key part of my life and the '51 Mercury. Those were important purchases in my life.

Interviewer: Have you always liked cars and I think motorcycles too?

George: I was coming to that. Motorcycles were [ ] cars[ ]. I was working up the ladder, but certainly motorcycles. The last two new ones were very, very nice motorcycles. I really enjoyed those.

Interviewer: Can you remember what age you were when you started to enjoy them?

George: Of those '98's, the one I bought last year, the '99, the one I bought in 1998, bought them both in 1998, one in the early spring and one in the [ ] and those were purchases. Of course, I guess the most important thing in my life was my marriage. Obviously that was prima. No question about that.

Interviewer: You were just saying your marriage was prima in your life.

George: Yeah that would be it. That would be the number one important item. That created the most trauma, so to speak. I worry about should I take on all these responsibilities. It probably shut me from getting around for at least a year. You know, whether I could do that or not. Whether I can handle the responsibility.

Interviewer: That is a big responsibility, especially when it is important. Had you and Shirley known each other for a long time?

George: A couple of years, which isn't long in today's terms, but it was back then. Yeah we took a lot longer than we do now. Before, you know, six months and you were done.

Interviewer: Are there other things that you would like to talk about as being important in your life or you remember as being important?

George: Well, it is all I can think of.

Interviewer: Are there roles that you have played in life that you feel good about, roles that you played either in your home, in the community or in the workplace? Are you finding it hard to concentrate on the questions?

George: Yeah I am tired, there is no question about that. How far do we have to go?

Interviewer: We only need to go as far as you feel up to going?

George: I don't know if I am ever going to feel more alert than I am.

Interviewer: Do you want to continue?

George: I think I would like to continue, but I find it difficult.

Interviewer: I am wondering maybe I will try a couple of different questions, but if you want to stop, please tell me to stop. Are there wishes or dreams for your family, for your kids, grandchildren, Shirley?

George: Yeah, sure there are. First of all I would like them to accomplish all the things that they want to do. Anything that I could have done in the past, of course it has passed, anything I can do now it would help them to accomplish that I would still like to do that. You know obviously all I can do is monetary, but I dearly would like to help them any way I could to capture what life experience or whatever would make their life better down the road.

Interviewer: Are there things that you would like to have your grandchildren know about their grandfather? Things you would like to say to them? . . . are you feeling you've had enough?

George: Yeah, I think so.

This example of Dignity Therapy is somewhat atypical. The patient is not only very sick, but he has too little energy to engage in detailed, rich responses, which are usually a part of Dignity Therapy. However, both he and his wife were anxious for him to take advantage of this opportunity, even if only in some small way. The final edited version of his transcript looked like this:

Interviewer: Can you tell me about your life, particularly the parts you remember as being the most important?

George: The purchase of new cars has always been an exciting thing for me over the years. Cars were an exciting thing to get involved in, and they gave me a good feeling. I remember one in particular, the '49 Mercury. It and the '51 Mercury are still a very key part of my life. Those were important purchases in my life. Motorcycles, too, were very important. The last two new ones were very, very, very nice motorcycles. I really enjoyed those.

Of course, I guess the most important thing in my life was my marriage to Shirley. Obviously that was prima. No question about that. That would be the number one important item. It created the most trauma as well. I worried whether I should take on all the responsibilities of marriage. That fear probably stopped me from getting around to marriage for at least a year. Could I do it or not? Could I handle the responsibility? Shirley and I had known each other for a couple of years, which isn't long in today's terms, but it was back then.

Interviewer: Are there wishes or dreams you have for your family, your kids, grandchildren, or Shirley?

George: There sure are. I would like them to accomplish all the things they want to. I can't help them out as I have in the past, but I would still like to help them to accomplish their goals, in any way I can. I feel all I can do is contribute in a monetary way now. But, I would dearly like to help them any way I could, to capture the life experiences that would make their life better down the road.

It is easy to see where the editorial changes have been made. In the basic cleaning up of the manuscript, partial sentences were either deleted (e.g., "Motorcycles were [] cars [] I was working up the ladder, but certainly motorcycles") or minor corrections were made to improve syntax ("A couple of years which isn't long in today's terms" becomes "Shirley and I had known each other for a couple of years, which isn't long in today's terms . . ." It is also easy to pick out content that was clearly not intended for the final generativity document; for example, "Well, it is all I can think of," or "Yeah I am tired, there is no question about that. How far do we have to go?" The interviewer's voice can be minimized in many instances; notice the interviewer's comments ("Do you know what made those important for you? Do you remember what made them important, the cars?" "Do you remember one in particular?" and "Have you always liked cars and I think motorcycles too?") have all been eliminated from the final document. Yet the responses to each of those questions appear in the final document as a concise paragraph, reading, "The purchase of new cars has always been an exciting thing for me over the years. Cars were an exciting thing to get involved in, and they gave me a good feeling. I remember one in particular, the '49 Mercury. It and the '51 Mercury, are still a very key part of my life. Those were important purchases in my life. Motorcycles too were very important. The last two new ones were very, very, very nice motorcycles. I really enjoyed those."

The final thing that George says in his actual interview, as a response to a question about feeling if he has had enough is, "Yeah, I think so." Clearly, this is neither an appropriate nor fitting ending to a document of such import. The editor/therapist chose a far more suitable way to conclude his generativity document: "I would dearly like to help them any way I could, to capture the life experiences that would make their life better down the road." This way, his final words are ones that express love and generosity for his family and look "down the road" toward their future.

While this example of Dignity Therapy may not be typical, George's family was pleased and moved by the results. Although he was very close to death, his wife was able to read it to him. At the conclusion of this reading, he said, "I was glad to be able to get that out." His wife, who died two years later, said that she read the document many times, and had given copies to his four children and their families. His wife said that her boys thought the transcript suited their dad perfectly; the things that were important to him included cars, motorcycles, and family. None of them had any problem with the order he chose to put these in.

6

FROM START TO FINISH

He who has gone, so we but cherish his memory, abides with us, more potent, nay, more present than the living man.

—Antoine de Saint-Exupery

Describing how to do Dignity Therapy—perhaps any kind of psychotherapy, for that matter—eventually begins to feel like the task of describing the taste of ice cream; no amount of description or carefully chosen assortment of adjectives quite captures the experience of having an actual taste. As much as I have tried to describe Dignity Therapy and all its complexities, readers may feel themselves, understandably, wanting to "have a taste." In teaching Dignity Therapy, there is no better way of providing this than by demonstrating an actual interview. Over the years I have had the privilege of conducting these demonstration therapy sessions in health care settings worldwide.

In China, I recall a patient who described how the Cultural Revolution had affected her and her family. I will always remember the Australian patient who, within days of dying, taught me that love and the wish to care for those dearest to us endures to our final days. Then there was a teaching session in eastern Canada, where a beautiful patient arrived at her Dignity Therapy session by wheelchair van from a local hospice—while her body, as she described it, "was broken," her spirit was very much strong and whole. Memories such as these are as numerous as are the many times I have demonstrated, before a group of health care professionals anxious to finally see with their own eyes, exactly how Dignity Therapy is done.

In this chapter, readers will find two examples of Dignity Therapy, verbatim, from start to finish. (Because of concerns regarding anonymity, both of these examples come from interviews done with simulated patients [professional actors]). The interviews were conducted in front of live audiences of health care providers during the course of two Dignity Therapy workshops. As with any patient, the interviews were not rehearsed or scripted in any way whatsoever. As per usual protocol, both patients received the Dignity Therapy question framework in advance of their actual interview. This provided them the opportunity to think about the questions and consider what content they might like to include in their Dignity Therapy.

Prior to starting the sessions, both patients answered a few questions that provided a *frame* for their Dignity Therapy sessions (see chapter 3). Readers are reminded that framing questions are usually quite brief and consist of contextual details such as patients' age, marital status, current living arrangements, whether they have children, their employment status, and some basic understanding of their current illness. The first case example took place at a 2008 palliative care congress in New Zealand. The patient identified himself as "Dave," a fifty-seven-year-old married man and father of three children—two daughters, Amy, age 18, and Kate, age 21, and a son, Will, age 24. Dave implied that his relationship with Will has not been easy for some time. Prior to being diagnosed with advanced colorectal cancer, Dave ran his own business doing outdoor landscaping.

DAVE'S DIGNITY THERAPY

Dr. Chochinov: OK Dave. How much of what you and I are about to do today has been explained to you?

Dave: Well I was told that if I, if I was willing, able, that you would, help me to kind of create a, a document, is that the word?

Dr. C.: Sure.

Dave: Yeah.

Dr. C.: Yeah.

Dave: To pass on to, people when I'm gone.

Dr. C.: That's right; for you to create something that might capture parts of you that you would want others to have.

Dave: That's right. Yeah. I mean I, I think that most of my family, people that are close to me probably know, stuff but, maybe there's, things of, that, that they don't know.

Dr. C.: OK.

Dave: Yeah.

Dr. C.: And it seems like the idea is something that must have had some appeal to you because, you decided to come here and do this.

Dave: Yeah. I, I, I don't, I'm like a lot of Kiwi blokes. I, I don't find it easy you know, know ta, talk about stuff.

Dr. C.: Well I'm just a Canadian bloke, so you're going to have to fill me in and tell me when things I'm asking don't quite work for you and when they do.

This comment is meant to make Dave feel that our time together should be comfortable and that at times, a certain amount of casualness and levity is perfectly appropriate.

Dave: Yeah.

Dr. C.: OK.

Dave: Yeah.

Dr. C.: Like everyone who does this Dave, I know you've been given a list of questions that we might choose to talk about. But I also want you to know that you are free to ignore those questions entirely. In fact, if there is anything that I ask of you, and you don't want to go there, just let me know you want to move onto something else.

Dave: Sure.

Dr. C.: I expect we will talk for about an hour, so if you are getting tired at any time, please, let me know. We have some water here for you; let me know if there is anything else you might need.

Dave: OK. Yeah.

Dr. C.: So how are you feeling about all of this?

Dave: I feel a bit nervous, talking about this. Some of it. As I say I'm not used to talking about, personal stuff.

Dr. C.: You seem a bit nervous. Is there anything that I might be able to do to help put your mind at ease?

Dave: Oh no it just. You're doing fine. Really.

Dr. C.: I hope so.

Dave: You know I, I'm starting to feel right. I mean I know that um, there are issues that I might feel, feel uncomfortable about, you know. But, m-most of the things in my life have been really, really good eh. You know. So if that's the kind of thing then, it's gonna be easy for me to do cause there's been a lot of good things.

Dr. C.: Dave, some people have specific ideas in mind about what they want to talk about. Is there a particular way that you want to do this, or like most people, would you prefer to have me help you get started and feed you questions along the way?

Dave: I, I prefer you to help me a bit. You know, like giving me questions.

Dr. C.: Perfect. So, before I turn on the tape recorder, let me remind you that the first question I will ask you is about recalling memories from your life that you might like to share.

Dave: OK.

Up until this point, the interview has primarily consisted of putting Dave at ease; being sure he understands the process fully and knows that he has compete control over what he will include, and what he chooses not to include. The tone of this introductory part of the interview should feel calm and the responses reassuring. Even though Dave will have had a prior explanation of Dignity Therapy, reviewing things that are unclear, clarifying any misunderstandings, and answering all questions is critical. If done well, this should help Dave anticipate what will happen during the interview and allow him to settle into it more easily.

> **Dr. C.:** The place I want to begin, Dave, is by having you tell me if there are memories you would most want to share or that you would most want remembered.

Communication skills are critically important in medicine, and this is no truer than when we are dealing with matters pertaining to life and death. Hence, exquisite attention must be paid to how clinicians choose their words. Words are a tool that can either help or harm, depending on how they are chosen and applied. Recall that when Dave is asked about his understanding of Dignity Therapy, he makes clear reference to passing on the document *when he is gone*. Dave's ability to articulate his situation in this direct fashion provides implicit permission to use similarly explicit vocabulary. "That you would most want remembered" is relatively explicit, in that it implies you will soon be gone. Had Dave used more euphemistic language or language avoidant of references to death (e.g. Dignity Therapy will let me share stories with people I love *or* Dignity Therapy should help me clear the air with my family), the therapist would need to be mindful of choosing words least likely to assault his healthy defenses. Had that been the case, the opening question might have been reshaped thusly: "The place I want to begin, Dave, is by having you tell me if there are parts of your life that you would most want others to know about." While these differences may seem subtle, they often make the difference between a comfortable and gentle interaction versus one in which the patient finds questions confrontational, grating, or even assaultive.

> **Dave:** There, there are yeah. There's a, there's a period of life. When Jean and I were first together, we weren't married, no kids.
>
> **Dr. C.:** So, so Jean is your wife?

Interrupting to obtain this kind of clarity is important. Unless the generativity document contains these personal details, there is the danger of it sounding rather generic. The difference between 'my wife' as opposed to 'Jean' helps ensure that

Dave's document is unique and specifically crafted for the benefit of those people he intends to leave it for.

> **Dave:** My wife yeah.
> **Dd. C.:** OK.
> **Dave:** Yeah. And we weren't married but, I've always been into the outdoors you know. I was doing, is able to do. I was, I was what you might call, a cruising hippy you know.
> **Dr. C.:** You know it sounds like fun. (slight chuckle) How old were you at this point?

Once again, obtaining this kind of information not only provides clarity in the document, but helps the interviewer to orient him or herself within the chronology of the particular story being told.

> **Dave:** Oh early twenties. We were both in our early to mid-twenties.
> **Dr. C.:** OK.
> **Dave:** And we had both been sailing the South Pacific. Hm.
> **Dr. C.:** I get the sense that as you nod your head, there are some particular memories or images that come to mind.
> **Dave:** Yeah.
> **Dr. C.:** If it isn't too difficult, would you be able to share some of those pictures that you are seeing in your mind's eye?

In Dignity Therapy, the metaphor of a photograph is often both useful and evocative. Applying this approach encourages patients to immerse themselves in their memories; connecting the memory to a concrete visual imagine often allows patients to describe the recollection more easily. Therapists can facilitate this process by enquiring about details contained within these pictures.

> **Dave:** Um. The, the people that I met, were, and in the islands, and actually the Solomon Islands particularly.
> **Dr. C.:** Right.
> **Dave:** And, they were, just, wonderful people. Um, and, and, I don't think that other people here in New Zealand who know me, uh, uh understand just quite what that period of my life was like.
> **Dr. C.:** This may be difficult, and may be even hard to articulate. As you were speaking, I noticed that you became rather tearful. Is there a particular image

that came to mind at that moment? If so, would you be able to describe it for me; and could you to describe it in as much detail as you recall?

This is a typical application of the photograph metaphor. Similar to clarifying the name of Dave's wife, eliciting a detailed description of his memories makes certain that the document is entirely unique. While others have visited the Solomon Islands, the inclusion of details ensures that only Dave could have produced this particular document. As such, in its uniqueness, the document conveys the inimitable life of its creator.

Dave: Um, uh the image would be the, uh of the village really and people. Uh almost like, you stepping out of a Polynesian exhibit from an Auckland museum.

Dr. C.: Um.

Dave: Where literally they're wearing very little but, the traditional grass skirt, and [ ] fresh from the dugout canoes and they, they live in houses that are, just thatch, and you know and so it's third world, it's a subsistence lifestyle that they live but, their values seem to me at the time to be, uh just fantastic, and I was very privileged just to be a part of their community, and, that photograph of me, being a part of their community uh I mean there's lots of shots really of, me a having the privilege of them, killing a pig for me. I know that sounds awful but that's a real privilege, killing a pig, it's a big deal. Um I helped to fix up their water supply. I put in wells at least. I didn't personally, but I gave them a lot of advice.

Dr. C.: Right. Right.

Dave: Of fixing up the water supply, which they had, cause otherwise, women were carrying, you know, dishes of water hours of their day. I created a tap. Yeah. Uh, just a tap. Um, I filled swimming pools and made that tap. That tap was much more use than the swimming pool.

Dr. C.: Absolutely. Again, I notice as you talk about it Dave, it seems a happy memory; but it seems to evoke a lot of emotion. Is that something that you wanted to talk about?

At this point, a cautionary note is in order. Pursuing affect is a technique common to most psychotherapies. It is often applied for the purpose of promoting insight, or more generally, to enable patients to take part in "uncovering" therapeutic work. In Dignity Therapy, however, following affect is a way of helping patients connect to their memories, thus eliciting the rich detail that will enhance their generativity document. This altered intent of pursuing affect can be an adjustment for many psychotherapists, who may need to shift their approach, so as not to derail Dignity Therapy by redirecting it toward an insight-oriented approach.

> **Dave:** Um. I suppose it's emotional just because, it was such a happy time.
>
> **Dr. C.:** Right.
>
> **Dave:** And *uncomplex*, you know simple, time, that uh, uh, I wish that more of my life could be like that.
>
> **Dr. C.:** Hm.
>
> **Dave:** My life kind of became more complex, when I started the business and I started employing people.

At this juncture, it was unclear whether shifting to his business dealings and the various complications this wrought was a selection of a "photograph" he wanted to share or simply him following a seemingly logical chronological pathway, having little to do with consciously choosing further content for purposes of generativity. To clarify this point, the photograph album metaphor was offered, allowing Dave to make a conscious choice about where to proceed next.

> **Dr. C.:** Maybe before we skip to that chapter of your life, people doing Dignity Therapy often imagine themselves sharing pictures in a photograph album with me. Now that you've shown me the photo of the Solomon Islands, are there others that come to mind, moments that you would want people to know about you, or to somehow be able to share?
>
> **Dave:** Yeah. Most of the photos would be to do with the outdoor type of thing cause that's, I guess, where I've had the best times. But in terms of a photograph of the early days, I would, I would again be involved with the Outward Bound Association. Cause I went there when I was a kid.
>
> **Dr. C.:** Right.
>
> **Dave:** And I'm part of the All Boys Association, and yeah a, a, a picture, well a series of pictures of me, climbing mountains and, doing rapids.
>
> **Dr. C.:** And again is this back in the Solomon Islands?
>
> **Dave:** No this is earlier. This is when I was younger really.
>
> **Dr. C.:** Well how old would you have been, and where was this picture taken?
>
> **Dave:** Eighteen. Um. Yeah. Down uh, Anakiwa, which is in the Marlborough Sounds and top of the south island.
>
> **Dr. C.:** Um-hum.
>
> **Dave:** Um, those, those photographs, though they were, they were, a very formative part of my life.
>
> **Dr. C.:** In what way?

Dave: Interest in the outdoors. Yeah. Yeah. Mind you, interest in the outdoors did occur before that as well with my father. My father ah, I was brought up rural community.

Dr. C.: And where abouts?

Dave: Farming. In what is now in what is almost part of Auckland.

Dr. C.: Um-hum.

Dave: And, ih, ma, ma, my dad was a farmer.

Dr. C.: Right.

DaveE: Um-hum. So. Yeah I mean farming and the outdoors was a part of my life.

By mentioning his father, early formative experiences and where he was brought up, it is clear that Dave's recollections are not organized around a strict chronology. He began his reminiscence by sharing a memory dating back to his early twenties. He then briefly mentions affiliating with the Outward Bound Association starting at the age of eighteen. So as not to lose the thread relating to his early upbringing, childhood recollections are, at this point, explicitly asked about.

Dr. C.: And is there a childhood image that emerges in your mind's eye as you talk about this, or is it more vague than that?

Dave: Oddly enough, it's not on the farm actually. Probably going on the golf course. Probably walking around to the edge, trying to toddle around after dad as cause he was a keen golfer.

Dr. C.: Oh really.

Dave: Yeah. Yeah. Very, very, very, very outdoor things.

Dr. C.: How old would you have been in that particular scene?

Dave: Four. Ha ha. Trying to be a caddy.

Dr. C.: Right. (slight chuckle)

Dave: Yeah. Yeah. Four. That, that was a, a probably formative part of my interest in the outdoors really. There were lots of beautiful pine trees big old ones. I loved the smell of pine needles ever since then.

Dr. C.: Um.

Dave: Yeah.

Dr. C.: This thread of the outdoors is something we can trace in each of the three images that you've shared, from the golf course, to the mountain climbing, to the Solomon Islands.

This particular comment is not meant to be interpretive. Rather, it is summative and is meant to illustrate to Dave that he is being carefully listened to, that his words matter and have totally captured the attention of the therapist.

Dave: Yeah. Yeah. It's all outdoor stuff.

Besides gently guiding the flow of the interview, the therapist must be mindful of timekeeping. Because of advanced illness, patients rarely have the energy to extend their session beyond one hour. As a general rule of thumb, the first half of the interview is devoted to personal memories and recollections. Having reached about twenty minutes into the interview, and Dave not having yet spoken of his wife, this seemed an appropriate opportunity to point him in that direction.

Dr. C.: It is. You mentioned that the Solomon Islands were where you and Jean also got together.

Dave: Yeah. We. We, we actually, um were together in New Zealand. We went away together. We were both. We met at a sailing club. We were both interested in sailing. And a, we got ourselves together, got ourselves a boat together, and we sailed to the Pacific, for three seasons, three glorious seasons really. Three seasons we did.

Dr. C.: I can't even begin to imagine what that must have been like.

Dave: Fantastic life style. Um.

Dr. C.: This may be difficult to put into words, this being such a large experience. You described it as a fantastic life style, extending over nearly three years of your life.

Dave: Yeah.

Dr. C.: Are there stories, memories, or images that you would want to speak to, or include as part of this?

Dave: Um. Certainly. Um, the top story is major, and for me putting the water supply in for the village people. Other stories, um being caught in a, in a nasty storm. Not life threatening but nasty, and, very uncertain cause it was before GPS. I was navigated by sexton. That's a lost art these days.

Dr. C.: Hm.

Dave: Satellite navigation um, and I was a bit uncertain. I'd done dead reckoning there were currents around, and there were reefs around, and I wasn't at all sure about quite where we were, and I mean I, I knew the basic facility, but I was concerned you've got the possibility of ending up on the reef. We were just trying to hold the position and, avoiding possibly landing up on a reef. And there was a canoe. I mean I was on a thirty-six-foot boat you know. I mean though she was a seaworthy boat. And there this little, I mean just a, it's something out of the Auckland Museum, and the, the sail was, you know was woven flat, and these people guided us. They, they had seen us. They were out fishing, going, "people what are you doing out there?"

Dr. C.: (slight chuckle)

Dave: But anyway they you know, hello, hello.

Dr. C.: (slight chuckle)

Dave: Where are we? Oh you know. You follow me kind of thing. Well actually when they came on board they tied up to me.

Dr. C.: Wow.

Dave: And, and they showed me the way, basically through this passage through this reef where I, I knew there was a reef, and I was worried about it. They showed me the passage, they knew, they were locals. And who did they save— me? What a spot.

Dr. C.: Extraordinary.

Dave: And I mean we, I was, we had been drifting around for, not well, not drift- ing, but, we had been at sea a couple of days at that point. And I was, really knackered, but just the feeling of having been, exhausted you know, salt encrusted and having being very worried. And the relief. These people guided me in. It was just absolutely, gorgeous anchorage. 360 degree protection. That's what one wants in protection, 360 degree protection just about and the storm outside.

Dr. C.: (slight chuckle) Um. Moving forward Dave. Almost reluctant to leave the 70s.

Dave: Yeah. Yeah.

Dr. C.: It sounds, spectacular.

Dave: It was spectacular.

Dr. C.: (slight chuckle) But moving forward, are there other images that follow. Again, if you and I were looking through that photograph album, what are the next ones that you would show that are important moments or chapters in your life?

Dave: Family.

Dr. C.: Tell me about that.

Dave: Well there have been so many people. Most people have had families. Um, regardless of the most important occasions of their lives. It certainly was with me.

Dr. C.: And when you say family, who are the people you are referring to?

Dave: Three kids. Will, first you know that's, and that's twenty-four years ago. First Will.

Dr. C.: Right.

Dave: Kate, a few years later. Amy. Um, yeah just having children was, uh, very, mind-boggling experience. First you're a young teenage bloke who, I mean I, I, I'd had brothers and sisters and everything so I was used to the whole family idea.

Dr. C.: Right.

Dave: And uh, but then my own family; that was fantastic. Yeah. And also, at that time I was actually, making a, a business go pretty well. So actually we were doing alright, it wasn't too much of a struggle.

Dr. C.: Hm. It sounds like for you, having family was a mind-altering experience.

Dave: It was.

Dr. C.: What took you by surprise? What made it so over the top amazing?

Dave: Having a, having a, baby boy, he was, it was, great. Baby. Kid. Things got harder actually. Um, as a little fella he was terrific. And as a baby a newborn baby he was gorgeous. I'll never forget. First baby you know. I mean, he was gorgeous. Total blond fella. He had blond hair. Oh dear. He was, he was the light of our lives you know. Um yeah the other two the other two, I mean Kate and Amy were also just equally as, as exciting to, hold when they came into the world. It was, yeah. I, I loved. Being a dad has been. Yeah. Its. It's been bigger than sailing.

Dr. C.: (slight chuckle). I guess what ties them together is the importance of safe harbors.

Dave: Yeah. Yeah. And also it's more challenging. Yeah.

Dr. C.: I'll bet.

Dave: Hm. I mean the girls are great. The girls have been good. I mean, Kate's in university. And she's probably gonna get into teaching like mum. Jean's a teacher, my wife.

Dr. C.: Right.

Dave: And she's probably go. She's thinking that she's doing education, go into teaching.

Dr. C.: And Amy?

Dave: Amy's good at school but she's good at science. She's thinking of doing physiotherapy maybe.

Dr. C.: And you've alluded to the fact that things with Will aren't quite so smooth. Is that something you had hoped to talk about in this document?

The friction that Dave alludes to between him and his son may or may not be something he wants to address in Dignity Therapy. Being an important family issue does not make it required content for Dignity Therapy. Ultimately, only Dave can determine what content must find its way into his therapy. In opening this up, however, one must be careful to monitor for, and if necessary manage, the so-called "ugly" stories—that is, content that might prove harmful to a generativity document recipient.

Dave: Yeah. Uh it was the thing I was probably most, um challenged by when I thought that, talking about the life you know. Talking about personal issues. It's talking about him. Yeah. Yeah kind of. Yeah. It's, it's not been easy lately. Hm. But I think I need to, say yeah I think probably, he's not even in the country, he's still in Paris. Thought he would have come back by now.

Dr. C.: You thought he would have come back by now, in view of . . . ?

Dave: Intuition. I mean we've only got a few months you know. Hm. He's come I think, he's just plain relived out his timing I reckon. I was hoping he would have come back by now.

Dr. C.: How long have things between you and Will been difficult?

Dave: A few years at least. Since university. He, he went to university.

Dr. C.: Right.

Dave: But he dropped out.

Psychotherapists new to Dignity Therapy sometimes feel torn between pursuing 'uncovering' lines of inquiry, versus adhering to a generativity agenda. This juncture in the interview represents a perfect example of when the novice Dignity Therapists may feel this very dilemma. At this moment of the interview, psychotherapists might feel inclined to pursue further detail about the nature of this conflict, to tease out the delicate and important interpersonal dynamics of this father-son relationship. On the other hand, the Dignity Therapist is ever mindful of the patient's story, and the need to facilitate the sharing of end-of-life reflections. However, one never wants to pursue the latter at the risk of seeming indifferent to the former. The skilled Dignity Therapist must find a way to acknowledge the implied, albeit vaguely described pain, while pointing out opportunities to inform generativity relevant content. The therapist tries to accomplish this in the follow way:

Dr. C.: People don't usually use Dignity Therapy to fix things that life has denied them the ability to sort out. But people often use Dignity Therapy to say things that they want said. Not that you're not going to have other opportunities to speak to Will, but if this is one chance for you to say to Will the things that you want him to know, what would you say?

Dave: Um. I'm sorry, for, being an asshole. Which I was. At times, a prick. I was a, authoritarian father figure. Uh, at a time when he didn't need that kind of thing. Dragged all the way down the hallway you know. Trying to bait me on. Say, you know, I wasn't gonna pay for the things he wanted. I was prepared to pay for his university, but I wasn't prepared to pay for other.

Dr. C.: Um.

Dave: So.

Dr. C.: So, would you like to say that you're sorry for the way you handled those things?

Dave: Yeah. It was a few years ago. Maybe a couple. Maybe. He was doing OK you know, in university and in, in assuming. He's a. He, he did a lot of outdoorsy stuff cause he, growing up. We were going to a ski club. He's a very good skier.

Dr. C.: Right.

Dave: But he's dropped away from that. Sailing of course. Although he wasn't. I always felt like I was pushing him a bit on that. Was a mistake.

Dr. C.: Hm.

Dave: Certainly kayaking he loved, stuff like that. But, he drifted away. He um, he wanted to become a street performer, a busker, basically. A clown. That's what he's doing. He's, he's at a place in Paris called Jacques Lecoq. It's a mime school.

Dr. C.: Hm.

Dave: And he's paying for it himself. Well. I'm not paying.

Dr. C.: You aren't paying, but it sounds like a part of you feels like you are paying.

Dave: I, I would have thought surveying would have been a great career you know. He was good at math and all that.

Dr. C.: Yeah. But you've taken a moment already to say, you're sorry for the way things went. Maybe sorry for decisions you've made. Again, this is your opportunity to add as many more words as you choose. Is there something else that you want Will to be able to hear directly from you?

Notice that these questions do not attempt to open up a full disclosure of what happened between Dave and his son. While Dave might have readily delved into details illustrating their painful past, it is unlikely that that would have served a useful purpose in terms of his Dignity Therapy. On the other hand, reminding him that this is a unique opportunity to create a record of things that need to be said moves him immediately toward taking a more conciliatory stance. Although the question, "Are there particular things that you feel need to be said to your loved ones, or things that you would want to take the time to say once again?" appears slightly later in the Dignity Therapy question protocol, introducing it at this point makes for a much smoother and less stilted interview.

Dave: That I still. Yeah I still love him. Even if he is gonna be a clown.

Dr. C.: (slight chuckle) The world needs clowns.

Dave: He, he is a natural comic. He's it naturally you know. I mean God, he's been working on the juggle you name it, he can do all that stuff. But now he's gonna,

gonna try make a career out of it you know. Hell. I'm trying. Its. Yeah. That career as being a clown, I, I could never stand that.

Dr. C.: Is it beginning to make any more sense with time, or are you simply learning to accept it?

Dave: Um. I think it's making sense more because, is why I, I was actually, thinking of him when I was thinking of the, the people on those Islands in the Solomon. There's a connection.

Dr. C.: Um-hum.

Dave: Uh. They wouldn't have minded if any of their sons wanted to be clowns. Although they'd still have to eat of course.

Dr. C.: Right.

Dave: Uh and he's got to eat yeah. But they, the, the simplicity I suppose about choices that those people have, is similar to the simplicity of choice that Will is making. And I think I've kind of come to understand that. I'd quite like a, I'd like to say a, to him that I understand his choice.

Dr. C.: I think you just did.

Dave: Yeah.

Dr. C.: Dave not meaning to rush you or push you ahead; you've shared a series of important images with me. Images that really capture some different periods in your life. Before we move on to other questions, are there any other pivotal images that you would hope to add to the collection?

Dave: Um. Getting, getting married to Jean. Um. Yeah she's been great. She's. I haven't wanted to be married to anybody else ever. Um but then I have said that to her you know and she does know that. But uh as an image, yeah the day that we got married um that's, that's pivotal.

Dr. C.: What do you see?

Notice again how effectively the picture metaphor evokes memories. The physicality of the metaphor allows the therapist to use concrete language—'what do you see'—to make the task of recollection so much more tangible for patients.

Dave: Um. Uh, outdoors again. We, we did get married on, on a boat.

Dr. C.: Surprise. Surprise. (chuckles)

Dave: Yeah. Yeah and then our honeymoon was the image is, is on, on the boat.

Dr. C.: And how old were you both?

Dave: Twenty-six um, um. Yeah. Uh and, uh yeah. She, she was a bit, twenty-five actually.

Dr. C.: Anything else before we move on?

Dave: Another formative pivotal pictures?

Dr. C.: Only if there are others that come to mind, which you feel important to share.

Dave: Um. There, there would be, um, pictures around home building. You know like first house. Uh and doing it up and then moving on, second house. Doing that up.

Dr. C.: Um-hum.

Dave: Yeah. Um. We've kind of grown out of that now. I'm sick of doing up houses.

Dr. C.: (slight chuckle)

Dave: We've done a few. But it, they are a great time as well you know.

Dr. C.: Right.

Dave: Yeah. Covered in paint. Whatever. Covered in cement. Yeah. But doing up, doing up homes. And there have been really important things, you know. As the, with the kids as well they've helped. Um-hum.

Dr. C.: I have a sense of how you might answer this, but are there particular roles and accomplishments that you feel most proud of?

This is the first time in the interview that the questions veer away from exclusively biographical inquiry. The first two questions in the Dignity Therapy protocol (see chapter 4) address life history and recollections to be shared with family members. The next two questions cover important roles, accomplishments and things the patient takes pride in. Dave has already addressed many of these issues to some degree. Because of time constraints and not having delved extensively into some of Dave's latter recollections, the question of roles, pride, and accomplishments was raised in order to provide another opportunity to elaborate on things he only touched on briefly. Not every question within the protocol needs to be asked of patients, as there is often overlap between them. These are decisions that therapists will need to make on a case-by-case basis, depending on how a particular Dignity Therapy session unfolds. Although one wants to create openings and opportunities for responses, this should be counterbalanced by avoiding what could be perceived as annoying redundancies.

Dave: Um the, the business. Yeah it's been really important because it's, it's supported us in our lifestyle. We've had a good life, and I, I have a partner now thank God, he can, he can take over this business you know and keep it going cause, because it's like. Yeah the business has been, something I'm proud of you know. It's a really good business. We do good quality work. Uh in a industry where there are gambles and, and you know. We don't build anything that falls over. Everything we build lasts. Yeah that's something I am really proud of you know. I can drive around this town, and I can see gardens that will be, around and like good for, fifty, a hundred years maybe, you know. Hopefully.

Dr. C.: So you take real pride in the quality and the sturdiness of your work.

Dave: I do. Yeah. Yeah. Yeah. You know.

Dr. C.: Hm.

Dave: And the way they're well designed too you know. Things fit in to um, with a, with, with um surroundings. Not. I mean, not big nasty places that, that don't look appropriate for the, for the space they're in. Um yeah. I'm not really a "greenie" but I suppose I am in a way. Yeah. Yeah.

Dr. C.: Are there other roles or accomplishments that you take particular pride in?

Dave: I work with the Out Bounders Association for young people. Out Bounders is a great association you know. Now I'm involved with that and I you know, I, I go to committee meetings and help fundraise. It's, it's a wonderful association for young people because these days, there more and more that they're helping other people, coping kids with you know, it's like kind of underprivileged kids.

Dr. C.: What makes that an important connection for you? I mean why that particular association?

This question was asked in order to demonstrate my careful attention and interest in his choice of Outward Bound. I also asked about the personal connection in order to individualize the rationale for this affiliation. As in other aspects of Dignity Therapy, questions that move the patient toward specific, detailed, and individualized answers add to the overall success of the generativity document itself.

Dave: Cause I went there when I was young and I'm helping keep the place going and keeping in financial, keeping with the fund raising events and so on. Uh and I and it's going strong, and I hope it continues to go strong. Because it does help a lot of people these days you know. In my day it was just well kind of not the privileged kids but, you had to have a few bucks to go there but these days a lot, a lot of people go there you know. I've thought it through and it starts people off in new directions. Yeah.

Dr. C.: Dave, besides those vocational and community roles you've shared, are there others? For example, what about family roles?

This question was purposely leading, in that while Dave had spoken extensively about his son and some of their troublesome issues, comments about his wife and especially his daughters have been quite brief. It is the role of the therapist to monitor these things, and attempt to create opportunities that might lead the patient to a rich, balanced, and overall complete Dignity Therapy.

> Dave: I've been a good Dad.
>
> Dr. C.: Can you talk about that?
>
> Dave: Well, I've all, I've always really enjoyed the um, the sideline Dad thing without trying to shout too much you know.
>
> Dr. C.: Right.
>
> Dave: But you know encouraged them along, always been there for them, trying to make time. Yeah. I mean cause it is hard when you're running a business and it's very tempting to say, oh I've got a meeting, I can't be there for that game. But I've tried to be there for the game and postpone the meeting and I've done that often.
>
> Dr. C.: So when you describe being a good Dad, can you put words to what that means to you?

As in other instances, this type of question is intended to draw Dave out of generalizations or platitudes, gently pushing him to describe his own perspective or experiences.

> Dave: Giving, well, well, to their needs and giving, the time, I think. If you can give them time, that's the thing I see most often. That, that are in my opinion, parents, often make the mistake of not giving their kids time. Just because they think the meeting is more important. You know the time for that meeting is more important than time for, standing on the sidelines and saying, you know, Run Amy Run, you know.
>
> Dr. C.: Right.
>
> Dave: Yeah.
>
> Dr. C.: And I think you have many recollections of saying "Run Amy Run" too.
>
> Dave: Yeah. Yeah. She is a good runner.
>
> Dr. C.: (slight chuckle)
>
> Dave: Yeah. Yeah. Yeah. That giving time, that's what I'm most proud of, I reckon.
>
> Dr. C.: Right.
>
> Dave: Cause that's not easy to do if you're busy.
>
> Dr. C.: Are there other recollections of fatherhood that come flooding back to mind?
>
> Dave: Um. Well birthdays of course, good, the good times, and the holidays. Cause yeah which we've, always been an active family you know. I, I mentioned

ski, ski club. We all, I'm not great but my kids are good. Uh, uh we're all local ski club members as well. I love getting down to the ski club. Yeah. Uh. Uh. Yeah. There is kind of experiences. The holiday experiences with your children.

Dr. C.: Um-hum.

Dave: You know there's so many good things that we've done. I wish I could take back some of the bad things that sometimes made their lives miserable.

Dr. C.: It sounds like given the chance, you would like to take that back or fix it; and you've begun to do that with some of the words you've shared with me here today.

The Therapist must be mindful that Dignity Therapy, while about the creation of a generativity document, is also about a "here and now" experience. Comments such as this show a deep empathic connection, which make the patient aware that he is being heard, and that his efforts and even his anguish are appreciated. This particular comment also affirms that what he has accomplished in his Dignity Therapy is powerful and possibly healing for the people he loves.

Dave: Um-hum.

Dr. C.:. Which leads me to another question. Are there things that you feel need to be said or you would like to take a moment to say, once again, to particular people in your life that matter to you?

Dave: Um. Well, my parents have gone but I've, I, I do have a brother who stayed running the farm.

Dr. C.: Um-hum.

Dave: I've never really said thanks to him because to be honest the, the farm subsidized me, a lot in the early days.

Dr. C.: What's your brother's name?

Dave: Bill.

Dr. C.: Bill.

Dave: Yes. Will and Bill.

Dr. C.: Right.

Dave: Will and Bill, a bit of a joke!

Dr. C.: I get it (slight chuckle)

Dave: A thank you cause he, he kinda. He's an older brother.

Dr. C.: Right.

Dave: And I don't really think he wanted to stay on the farm. Neither of us did. But he was loyal to the old man and stayed on the farm and I think that I owe him a thanks because he kinda subsidized me in my early life.

Dr. C.: Hm.

Dave: And. I, you know now I should be. I, I kind of dropped out of sight in those days, those hippie kind of days if you like. While he was, keeping the farm going.

Dr. C.: OK.

Dave: And I don't think he, deep down, knew whether he wanted to, I think he was jealous, not jealous, he is a little bit, the fact that I took off and he stayed on.

Dr. C.: And are there other people that you have things specifically that you would like to say or to take the moment to say once again?

Dave: And I've got two sisters, too. I, I've never said thanks for their support.

Dr. C.: And their names are?

Dave: I need to thank Jean. I've never, I've never, I've never thanked people enough really you know. My partner as well. Wayne's great. There's so many people I've never said thank you and I always just kind of, I, I, been too busy getting on.

Dr. C.: So I hear you say thank you to Wayne.

Dave: Yeah he's my partner because he's been a great business partner.

Dr. C.: And you were starting to say something to your sisters.

Dave: Yeah. Yeah. Linda yeah she's a older sister as well.

Dr. C.: Um.

Dave: She, she told me a lot. My sister. About just, um, I think probably you would call it respect for other people really. She is a really, really good person. A really good person. Social worker. She's always concerned about other people. And she, uh has taught me to be less selfish than I might have been inclined to be. Yeah.

Dr. C.: And your other sister?

Dave: Yeah. She yeah she's lovely. Younger sister, baby really.

Dr. C.: And I'm sorry her name is?

Dave: Oh we call her Poochie.

Dr. C.: Poochie.

Dave: Her name is Patricia. Pat.

Dr. C.: Right.

Dave: Pooch.

Dr. C.: (slight chuckle)

Dave: But anyway. Yeah she's just like the little, you know, the favorite little baby sister.

Dr. C.: Right.

Dave: Yeah. Yeah. She, she always makes me laugh. She's. Maybe that's, she, she's always been into kind of, into dramatics. Um maybe that's where Will gets it. Maybe it runs in the family through her.

Dr. C.: Now what about your immediate family? We've talked a little bit about Jean. We've talked a little bit about your three children; perhaps many of these things, you feel you've already said. But given the opportunity to say something or to take the time to say something once again, what do you hope each of them might hear?

Dave: Um. That I've always. Um. That I've always, in my own I, I've always loved them in my own funny kind of way you know. That I haven't maybe been able to say that. I'm, I'm, it's a, I'm, I, it's funny with Jean, I've always been able to, tell her that I've loved her but, not the rest of my family.

Dr. C.: Hm.

Dave: It's not something I've been able to say. I've never been able to say that to my brother, or my sisters. Or, or to Will. I have, I have been able to do the girls, but not to Will.

Dr. C.: I heard you mention it earlier, and I just heard you tell them all again that you love them.

Dave: Yeah.

Dr. C.: Is there something you need to add to that?

Dave: I think that I did say before to Will that, but that I'm, that I'm sorry. For being um, bit of a, dictatorial prick at a time when I don't think he needed that. He needed more understanding in me.

Dr. C.: Hm.

Dave: Um when he was chasing a different path. You know just because he wanted to become a clown, and I wanted him to be a surveyor. I mean. Yeah.

Dr. C.: Dave. None of us know how much time we have. None of us know exactly the number of our days. But, in thinking about the future, and in helping them to prepare for a future that you might not be a part of, are there words of advice, or instruction that you would want to leave with them to somehow help them with whatever lies ahead?

The question regarding hopes, wishes, and dreams for loved ones is often very poignant and elicits wonderful and meaningful responses. However, given that Dave had just expressed his deep feelings of love for his family and asked his son for forgiveness—and we were reaching the end of our time together—I selected to ask a question regarding final words of advice or instructions. This question felt more consistent with the previous questions regarding what needed saying, and seemed a smoother transition toward a closing of this therapeutic session.

Dave: Make time for other people. Uh. And, live every day like it's your last.

Dr. C.: Hm.

Dave: Um. Yeah make the days count. Really make them count. Yeah. Especially I say that to Will. Yeah. Life can be short. Yeah. And, it's a, it's kind of a biblical saying I suppose. But, you know, be good to other, do to other people what you know, you'd only do to yourself.

Dr. C.: These sound like very thoughtful and wise pieces of advice.

Dave: Um. It's the, the people on islands in the Solomons. It's how they lived. Yeah. And they had nothing. They had nothing. Hm.

Dr. C.: It sounds like you took in a lot of their advice, and perhaps lived your life in some ways, being guided by that very advice.

Dave: Yeah. Hm. Yeah. Cause I haven't, I mean I haven't always done that you see.

Dr. C.: Dave, is there anything more you want to say before I shut off the audio recorder?

Dave: No, I think I've done what I came here to do. You can shut it off now.

Chapter 5 provides a detailed description of how Dignity Therapy editing is to be done. However, seeing an entire, raw transcript transformed into a complete generativity document can be enlightening and makes the process so much more tangible. Much of the opening of Dave's transcript was deleted, as it largely provided demographic information about his children that was easily later incorporated into the document. His sentence, "I'm like a lot of Kiwi blokes . . ." opens the edited transcript, as it seems a fitting start for Dave's generativity document.

DAVE'S GENERATIVITY DOCUMENT

Dr. Chochinov: Dave, can you tell me about your life, particularly the parts you remember most or think are most important?

Dave: I'm like a lot of Kiwi blokes; I don't find it easy to talk about *stuff*. There's a period in my life, like when Jean, my wife and I, were first together. We weren't married and didn't have kids. I was what you might call a *cruising hippy*. Jean and I were both in our early to mid twenties at the time. We met at a sailing club in New Zealand and went away together. We were both interested in sailing and got ourselves a boat together. We sailed in the Pacific for three years. Fantastic life style.

Italics and boldface type can be used sparingly, in the written document, to give the reader a sense of where the patient has placed emphasis, e.g. "stuff" and "cruising hippy." Italics imply soft emphasis while boldface implies strong emphasis. The words "like when" would not be used in more formal style of speaking, but are part of Dave's particular style and make the voicing distinctly his.

> We met people in the Solomon Islands particularly, who were just wonderful. I don't think that other people here in New Zealand, who know me, understand quite what that period of my life was like. An image from that time that comes to mind would be of a village and the people who lived there. It was almost like stepping into a Polynesian exhibit at the Auckland museum. The people were wearing very little but the traditional grass skirt. They lived in houses that were just thatch. It was a third world, subsistence lifestyle, but their values seemed to me, at the time, to be just fantastic. I was very privileged to be a part of their community. I felt I was a part of their community. There was the privilege of them killing a pig for me. I know that sounds awful, but that's a real privilege, killing a pig. It's a big deal. I put in wells for them—well I didn't personally, but I gave them a lot of advice. I helped to fix up their water supply by creating a tap, just a tap, because women were carrying containers of water for many hours of their day. I have built swimming pools, but that tap was of much more use than a swimming pool. The tap story and helping to put in the water supply is major.

Some of the words in the original transcript may not be clear—e.g. the Solomon Islands was originally transcribed as "Saltzman Islands"; it is important to get the right name and spelling.

> Talking about this time is emotional for me because it was such a happy, uncomplex, simple time. I wish that more of my life could be like that. My life became more complex when I started the landscaping business and employing people.
> Another picture that comes to mind around that time is being caught in a nasty storm. Not life threatening, but nasty and very uncertain because it was before GPS. I was navigating by sexton, which is a lost art these days. I knew that there were currents and reefs around, but I wasn't at all sure quite where, and I was worried about it. What a spot! I knew the basics, but I was concerned, because you've got the possibility of ending up on the reef. We were just trying to hold the position and avoid the possibly of landing up on a reef.
> We had been at sea a couple of days at that point, and I was exhausted, salt encrusted and very worried. There I was, on a thirty-six-foot seaworthy boat and then, out in the sea, I saw this little boat, something that could have come out of the Auckland Museum, with the sail woven flat. These two people were

out fishing on this canoe-like boat, and had seen us. I am sure they were thinking, "People, what are you doing out there?" When they came on board, they
tied up to me and showed me a passage through the reef. They were both
locals and knew where the passage was. These two people saved me! The relief!
These people guided me in to an absolutely gorgeous anchorage, with 360
degree protection. That's what one wants—360 degree protection with the
storm outside. It was spectacular.

Dave's words on page 126 of the original transcript have been added to those he
shared at the beginning of the interview; they fit together chronologically, enhance
the picture he is describing, and help the transcript to read as prose as opposed to
dialogue. The conversation on pages 126 and 127 has been condensed, eliminating
the words of the therapist.

Dr. C.: Are there other special moments that you would want to talk about?

Dave: Most of the times would be to do with outdoor types of things, because I
guess that's where I've had the best times. In the early days I was involved with
the *Outward Bound Association*. I went there when I was a kid and I'm now
part of the *All Boys Association*. When I was younger, about eighteen, I would
have been climbing mountains and doing rapids. Those times were a very formative part of my life, in terms of an interest in the outdoors.

An interest in the outdoors did occur before that as well, with my father. I was
brought up in a rural, farming community, in what is now almost part of
Auckland. My dad was a farmer, so farming and the outdoors was a part of my
life. Oddly enough, what I remember most is not on the farm actually. It's
walking around to the edge of a golf course, trying to toddle around after dad,
because he was a keen golfer. I was about four years old then, trying to be a
caddy! There were lots of beautiful big, old pine trees on that golf course.
I have loved the smell of pine needles ever since. That was probably another
formative part of my interest in the outdoors.

Dr. C.: Are there other important memories Dave?

The demographic information provided at the beginning of the interview, regarding names and ages of children, has been added to the section below where Dave
talks about his family.

Dave: I have three kids. Amy's eighteen, Kate's twenty-one, and Will is
twenty-four. Just having children was a very mind-boggling experience. First
I was a young teenage bloke, and then I had my own family! I had brothers and

sisters, so I was used to the whole family idea, but *my own* family was fantastic. At the time Will was born, the business was doing all right, and it wasn't too much of a struggle, so having a baby boy was great. However, things got harder with him actually. As a little fella, Will was terrific, and as a new born baby he was gorgeous. I'll never forget—our first baby. He was gorgeous and had blond hair. He was the light of our lives.

In the unedited transcript, Dave had said, "First you're a young teenage bloke who, I mean I, I, I'd had brothers and sisters and everything so I was used to the whole family idea. And uh, but then my own family; that was fantastic." In order to allow the narrative to read more easily, the sentence was reorganized to read as follows: "First I was a young teenage bloke and then I had my own family!"

Talking about Will was the thing I was probably most challenged by, when I thought about taking part in this interview, and talking about personal issues. It's not been easy lately. He's in Paris. I was hoping he would have come back by now. Things have been difficult between us for a few years at least, since he dropped out of university.

Dr. C.: Are there things that you would want to say to Will?

Dave: I'm sorry for being an asshole, which I was and at times I was a prick. I was an authoritarian father figure, at a time when he didn't need that kind of thing. A few years ago, I would say I wasn't going to pay for the things he wanted. I was prepared to pay for his university, but I wasn't prepared to pay for other things.

The words "asshole" and "prick" might sound jarring; however, they are words that Dave chose and thought fitting. Once Dave hears or reads the edited document in its entirety, he would have an opportunity to remove these words, should he so choose. They are not, however, part of an "ugly story," in that they will not be interpreted as assaultive, but rather, help articulate a clear and sincere apology.

He did a lot of outdoorsy things growing up. He's a very good skier, but he's dropped away from that. I always felt I was pushing him a bit on that. That was a mistake. Certainly he loved kayaking and stuff like that, but he drifted away. He wanted to become a street performer, a busker basically, a clown. That's what he's doing at Jacques Lacoq mime school in Paris. He's paying for it himself. He was good at math, and I would have thought surveying would have been a great career.

I still love him, even if he is going to be a clown. He's a natural comic, but now he's going to try to make a career out of it. Hell, I'm trying! A career as a clown!

I could never understand that. But I think it's making more sense now. I was thinking of him when I was talking about the people in the Solomon Islands. There's a connection. They wouldn't have minded if any of their sons wanted to be clowns, although they'd still have to eat of course. But the simplicity I suppose, in the choices that those people have made is similar to the simplicity of the choice that Will is making. I think I've come to understand that. I'd like to say to him that I understand his choice.

These words about Will were combined from the narrative on page 127-131 and page 137.

The dialogue reads, "But they, the, the simplicity I suppose about choices that those people have, is similar to the simplicity of choice that Will is making." A slight revision makes the sentence so much easier to read and understand. "But the simplicity I suppose, in the choices that those people have made is similar to the simplicity of the choice that Will is making."

Dr. C.: Can you talk about the memories you have of your daughters?

Dave: Kate and Amy were equally as exciting to hold when they came into the world. I loved being a dad. It's been bigger then sailing! Also, it's more challenging. The girls are great. Kate's in university, and she's probably going to get into education and then teaching like her mum. Amy's good at school and science. She's thinking of doing physiotherapy next year.

Dr. C.: Are there other important times that you would add to those you've already shared?

Dave: Getting married to Jean. She's been great. I haven't wanted to be married to anybody else, ever. I have said that to her, and she does know that. The image of the day we got married—that's pivotal. It was in the outdoors again on a boat. When I think about our honeymoon, I think about being on the boat. Jean was twenty-five, and I was twenty-six.

Then there would be building our home. Doing up our first house and then moving on to the second house and doing that up. I'm sick of doing up houses! We've grown out of that now. But they were great times. Covered in paint and cement, doing up homes. There have been other really important times with the kids as well.

Dr. C.: Are there things you have accomplished in your life that have been important to you Dave?

Dave: The business is something I've been proud of. It's been really important, because it's supported us in our lifestyle. We've had a good life, and I have a very good business partner—Wayne—thank God. He can take over this business and keep it going. It's a really good business in an industry where there are gambles. We do good quality work, and we don't build anything that falls over. Everything we build lasts. That's something I am really proud of. I can drive around this town and see gardens that will be around for another fifty, maybe a hundred years. And they're well designed to fit in with the surroundings. Not big nasty places that don't look appropriate for the space they're in. I'm not really a "greenie," but I suppose I am in a way!

In the unedited dialogue, the interviewer provides a summative comment: "So you take real pride in the quality and the sturdiness of your work too." Although Dave does not specifically say "The business is something I've been proud of," he does affirm the therapists statement in various ways. "Everything we build lasts"; "And they're well designed to fit in with the surroundings. Not big nasty places that don't look appropriate for the space they're in" both exemplify his pride. Not often, but on occasion, the editor might incorporate something said by the interviewer—and very clearly affirmed by the patient—if doing so seems particularly important and not stated elsewhere in the patient's own words.

I am also proud of the work I do at the Outward Bound Association for young people. It's a wonderful association for young people, because these days, more and more, they're helping underprivileged kids to cope. It's an important place to me, because I went there when I was young. In my day you had to have a few bucks to go to the club, but these days a lot of people go there who don't have much money. I'm helping to keep the place going with the fundraising events and committee meetings. It's going strong, and I hope it continues, because it does help a lot of people these days. I think it starts people off in new directions.

The use of colloquialisms (e.g. "bucks") need not always be eliminated, as they can help capture the speaker's authentic and distinctive voice.

I've been a good Dad. I've always really enjoyed the sideline Dad thing, without trying to shout too much. I encouraged the kids along, and have always been there for them, trying to make time for them. It is hard when you're running a business and it's very tempting to say, "Oh I've got a meeting, I can't be there for that game." But I've tried to be there for the game and postpone the meeting. I've done that often. I think being a good dad means giving to the kids' needs and giving the time. I think parents often make the mistake of not giving their kids time, just because they think the meeting is more important than time on the sidelines saying, "Run Amy Run." *By the way, Amy is a good runner!* That—giving time—that's what I'm most proud of, because that's not easy to do if you're busy. We've always been an active family. I mentioned the ski club. I'm not a great skier, but my kids are good. Those kinds of experiences are important, like the holiday and birthday experiences with your children. There are so many good things that we've done and good times that we've had.

Although the interviewer asked several questions regarding accomplishments and important connections in the three preceding pages of dialogue, it is not necessary to include the interviewer's voice repeating them all. The initial question, "Are there things you have accomplished in your life that have been important to you Dave?" allows the narrative to flow easily—even if there is more than one idea identified.

Although some might leave out the phrase, "By the way, Amy is a good runner," the editor thought it added a nice and rather playful touch to the document.

Dr. C.: Are there things that you would like to take a moment to say, or say again, to people in your life who matter to you?

Dave: There are so many people I've never said thank you to. I've been too busy getting on. I've never thanked people enough really. My parents have gone, but I do have an older brother, Bill, who stayed on running the farm. I've never really said thanks to him, because to be honest the farm subsidized me a lot in the early days. I don't really think he wanted to stay on the farm. Neither of us did. But he was loyal to the old man and stayed on. I think that I owe him thanks, because he subsidized me in my early life. I kind of dropped out of sight in those days, those hippie days if you like, while he was keeping the farm going. I don't think he knew deep down, whether he wanted to. I think he was a little bit jealous of the fact that I took off, and he stayed on.

I've got two sisters too. I've never said thanks for their support. Linda, my older sister, taught me a lot about respect for other people. She is a really, really good person. Linda is a social worker, and she's always concerned about other people. She has taught me to be less selfish than I might have been inclined to be. My younger sister, Patricia or Pat is lovely. We call her "Poochie." She's the favorite little baby sister. She always makes me laugh. Poochie has always been into dramatics, and maybe that's where Will gets it. Maybe it runs in the family through her!

I've always loved my family in my own funny kind of Kiwi way, but I haven't always been able to say that. It's funny with Jean. I've always been able to tell her that I've loved her, but not the rest of my family. I've never been able to say that to my brother or my sisters. Somehow it's been easier with the girls, but not with Will.

The interviewer's words, "I heard you mention it earlier, and I heard you tell them that you love them" are not used. Instead, the participant's words, "I've always loved them in my own funny way" are much more authentically "Dave."

> **Interviewer:** Dave, are there words of advice or instruction that you would want to leave with your family, to somehow help them with whatever lies ahead?
>
> **Dave:** Make time for other people. Live every day like it's your last. Make the days count, really make them count. I haven't always done that you see. Life can be short. The people on the Solomon Islands had nothing, and that's how they lived. It's kind of a biblical saying I suppose, but do to other people what you'd do to yourself.

This certainly provides a suitable and dignified ending. Appropriate endings might be found anywhere in the transcript. However, they often appear toward the end of the interview after the questions regarding "words of advice" and "wishes or dreams" are raised.

Dave does say in the transcript, "Really make them count. Yeah. Especially I say that to Will." The editor did not include that particular sentence; this could later be raised with Dave, to see if he did in fact want that included, or whether he might think that could be hurtful for Will to read and perhaps not understand the context.

Notice throughout the final edited document that grammar and punctuation are not entirely perfect or formal. The goal in editing should be to try and capture the fashion in which the participant uses speech and language. Also note that the original nineteen-page transcript is now a seven-page document. Yet it reads so much more clearly and coherently, and throughout, so transparently and authentically "Dave."

BILL'S DIGNITY THERAPY

Bill is a sixty-nine-year-old gentleman with end-stage cancer; he has been told, and seems to appreciate, that he has only a few months left to live. He and his wife, Janet, have been married for forty-five years and have three children: Donna, age forty-five; Ed, age forty-two; and David, age forty. He has five grandchildren including eighteen-month-old Cole, five-year-old Jack; Lindsay, who is eleven; Dorie, who is thirteen; and Samantha, who is eighteen years old. Until he got sick, Bill had been working as an accountant.

(This interview took place in Spring of 2010, at the first International Dignity Therapy Symposium held in Winnipeg, Canada)

(Tape recorder on)

Dr. Chochinov.: OK Bill. Maybe we can start by you telling me a little bit about your life. Particularly things that you think were important or things you would want known by your family.

Bill: Well I, I, I guess, one, does look back on their life when, you confronted with all of this.

Dr. C.: Hm.

Bill: Um, I'm not sure what kind of a exciting life I've left, lead, but the, I mean the, I was in accounting for, a number of years and then went into a, a consulting, with my own company, that type a thing. And . . .

At this early point in the interview, it felt important to get oriented to the chronology of Bill's story. Thus, the following question was asked.

Dr. C.: How old would you have been when you started into accounting?

Bill: Oh that was, pretty soon after school ya know. Yeah uh, I was uh, around twenty I guess when I went, went into accounting. Yeah.

Dr. C.: And so by age twenty, you had completed your training as an accountant.

Bill: I went for some training and uh, uh um uh, and then I, I went for um, became a chartered accountant, and um, um by the time, I got uh married, uh, I, was an accountant.

Dr. C.: And how old were you when you got married?

Bill: Twenty-four.

Dr. C.: So this was a pretty important time in your life, finding a vocation and moving into marriage.

Bill: Yeah. It, wasn't something we planned. That's for sure. It just happens you know. When you're young you don't, there's not much thought of the future. It's just, what you're doing now.

Dr. C.: I understand.

Bill: And uh, so yeah we, when we got, married it was a, um, uh, well the most important thing that happened to me at that stage of my career. The rest would have been children. That would have been the next thing.

Dr. C.: Of course.

Bill: Uh, uh, um, at that, that had any kind of meaning. Accounting is not a very, exciting career. It's pushing paper around.

Dr. C.: But Janet was more exciting.

Bill: Well, I sorta lucked out with her you know, cause she uh, she went along with my particular, dreams and chasing things.

Dr. C.: Hm.

Bill: And uh, that um, uh I don't know, imagine we had, we had Donna right off the bat too.

The rather vague and sweeping responses that Bill provides are not atypical of someone who is feeling unwell and has limited energy. Large swaths of history are presented in ways that are exceedingly brief and nondescript. At at this point, the questions move towards eliciting far more detail on important issues.

Dr. C.: Maybe we could just back up for a moment. You were talking about meeting Janet, and I'm wondering if you can tell me how that happened?

Bill: Well actually, we belonged to the uh same church. That's how, that's where we met, and it was through different socials at the church that we started to go around together.

Dr. C.: Right.

Bill: And um, we uh, um, first time I went out with her really I, I invited her and another girl at the same time (slight chuckle) to a party.

Dr. C.: That sounds exciting.

Bill: Uh yeah that was exciting that, the um, that, the um, it ended up the other girl, um, didn't take too kindly to that, and so Janet, was there (slight chuckle) and that's how we, basically got going around together.

Since Bill just mentioned meeting his wife, the photograph metaphor was as a way of encouraging him to provide some further details or additional related anecdotes.

Dr. C.: Bill, let's imagine that you and I are looking through a photograph album of your life, and you have just opened up the album on a page with a picture labeled "meeting Janet." Can you tell me what that photograph looks like?

Bill: I remember trying to neck with her. That was a, yeah that was uh, that was a big thing for me (slight chuckle) in a way.

Dr. C.: Were you nervous, were you frightened?

Bill: Not. No not at that stage. I just, wanted to neck. (slight chuckle) I had to think whether the, you know, the, take that to another step. But we did start going around together when, uh we would uh, uh when I was driving her home, we'd park outside of her house, and of course we'd, do some necking there, and uh, until her mother would come a flip the switch on. It was time to come in, you know so, that I remember.

Dr. C.: It sounds like there was a connection between the two of you. What was it about Janet that made you "see yourself as being lucky?"

Bill: I guess there was um, finding somebody, that I, I never had in my life, in my, uh, it was, it was just finding somebody you know, that was missing.

Dr. C.: And did you have a way of knowing that she was the missing piece; that this was someone who could fill that space?

Notice how the therapist uses the patient's language, thus showing that he is an attentive listener and in synch with Bill's story.

Bill: I didn't know that at the time. I mean really the, the, it was just the, um, you know total attraction. I mean I didn't analyze it that way. But looking back on it, I didn't know there was something missing in my life and um, and she certainly filled that uh, that void.

Dr. C.: And do you remember coming to the realization that this will be my life partner?

Bill: You know the, it wasn't uh something that clicked and that turned around and said you know.

Dr. C.: Yes.

Bill: It wasn't that; it was just, something it was like we were going around, and all of a sudden it was like, well, let's get married.

Dr. C.: Hm.

Bill: You know and uh, uh um, the, the, you know we talked about children and things like that but it was uh, it, it just wasn't a light bulb that went on. It was just something that we grew together. Um and then, and it's been that way basically ever since.

Dr. C.: You've continued to grow together.

Bill: Yeah. Yeah. Not that she hasn't wanted to kick my ass once in a while, but you know, but still, she was uh. That's what basically happened yeah. I, I, I, I don't understand people when then say um you know love at first sight and all that sorta stuff. Uh it certainly wasn't with me. Um, but it's like I've never been without her.

Dr. C.: Maybe I've asked this already, but were there things about Janet that drew you to her; perhaps something about her way of being?

Again, the therapist is attempting to elicit more detail regarding Bill's recollections of Janet and their early relationship.

Bill: Well, we're opposites, you know.

Dr. C.: (slight chuckle) Those sometimes mesh very well.

Bill: Her, her personality, apart from being very, wanting to be very organized and.

Dr. C.: Right.

Bill: And taking care of things and, and that kind of thing. But her personality was one of um, uh laughter, and I remember, that, it, it was just, and, and her whole family was the same way. Her whole family. She was the oldest of eight children, and, living in a small house really, but that house was, a joy to go to. It was fun. It always was and she, she had that, that she took that.

Dr. C.: Right.

Bill: And that's sort of. . . . apart from her mother's cooking that's the other, the other thing was her personality.

Dr. C.: Right. When you talk about that small house and, being filled with laughter, I sense that your mind takes you back to that place, that perhaps you can picture what it was like to be there in those fun moments.

Bill: Well yeah I, uh the, because it was such a different family than mine.

Dr. C.: So if you think back to that time, is there a particular image or photo that you find yourself looking at . . . being in Janet's, laughter filled home?

Bill: I think about being in the kitchen.

Dr. C.: The kitchen.

Bill: Sure.

Dr. C.: What do you see? What's happening?

Bill: Everybody gathered there.

Dr. C.: What's the occasion?

Bill: It didn't matter. Ev, every occasion, it, ev everybody ended up in the kitchen.

Dr. C.: Right.

Bill: You know when you get that large a family, standing around at a kitchen, and laughing, you know that's, that's what I remember.

Dr. C.: Right.

Bill: Yeah.

Dr. C.: So it's not a particular occasion, it's just every occasion.

Bill: Yeah. I remember Sunday dinners. We always used to go over there for Sunday dinner.

Dr. C.: And what was that like?

Bill: Again it was always, it was everybody crammed in that kitchen, laughing and having a good time.

Dr. C.: And what were you laughing about?

Bill: Anything. Anything and everything. Anything and everything. And it was uh, . . . her mother died, of cancer, and um, um ih, the, it's one thing I said at the funeral, I always remember the house with laughter. Hm. And that's I still do, the house is still there. Her dad still lives in the house. I, that's the, the way that house is remembered. With laughter.

Dr. C.: It sounds like a lot of beautiful memories there.

Bill: In that house there was, yeah.

Given that Bill started his Dignity Therapy by recalling times dating back to his early 20's, the therapist at this point attempts to explore whether there are earlier memories that he might wish to address.

Dr. C.: Yeah. Turning back a few pages in this album, you mentioned that your own life was very different than Janet's life. Are there some earlier memories or earlier photographs that you and I might glance at?

Bill: Well, ih, my upbringing wasn't the, the happiest of upbringings so it, the memories that I have are um, are short. Um the mainly because the other memories I don't really ih, dwell on, you know so that, the uh, I remember things like, the old car, actually a Model T Ford. I remember that. Now my brother's got it.

Dr. C.: (slight chuckle) How old were you in that memory?

Bill: Oh I was, just I kid. I was ten, twelve years old.

Dr. C.: And you remember the car well?

Bill: I remember the car. I remember two cars.

This is a perfect opportunity to have Bill engage in a memory by inviting him to recount as much detail as possible.

Dr. C.: Tell me about them. What do you remember?

Bill: Well, I remember my brothers. Ih, they, they went together and bought, ah the car, the one car. We used to have a field next to our house, and they used to park the car out in the field and stand around like a bunch of peacocks you know, strutting their stuff because they had a car.

Dr. C.: (slight chuckle)

Bill: But they uh, uh, I remember them. I can see them, totally standing there you know, my big brothers. I was the youngest of five brothers, five boys. Uh and they uh, they just um, uh there's things like that, there's things around the field. There's, where we used to play ball in the field, that kind of thing. Those kind of things I remember. I remember my dog.

Dr. C.: What was your dog's name?

Bill: Skippy. Yeah. He was uh, a cocker spaniel. You know. I don't even think that dog was, was the first dog that was really ours. It was our neighbors, but we inherited it.

Dr. C.: Right.

Bill: We stole it. (slight chuckle)

Dr. C.: (slight chuckle)

Bill: And uh, but I had another dog which was Prince, which was a uh, uh cross between an Irish setter and a black lab. That was my pal. You know. And they had to, after we got married they, they had to put the dog down so.

Dr. C.: Hm.

Bill: Yeah, that was sort of an end of an era for me and beginning of a new one, you know.

The therapist doesn't want to give Bill's childhood short shrift by avoiding it entirely (in view of Bill having said that this was an unhappy time in his life). Therefore, the comment that follows is important, in that it offers Bill choice about how he might proceed.

Dr. C.: Of course. Bill, you suggested that there are a lot of things about those early years—and those early photographs—that you don't particularly want to talk about. And I think I told you earlier today that this needs to be about you. So if there are things that you would just as soon not look at, we don't need to. But if there are things that you want to recount or you think important to share, this would be the time to do it.

Bill: Well it's just that I came from such a different family than, than what Janet. A, a totally, dysfunctional in many respects and not a very happy family.

Dr. C.: Hm.

Bill: Uh, and I guess maybe even wanting to get married, it was part of my escape from that, even though I was twenty-four at the time, and I was still living at home, even though I didn't like, living at home.

Dr. C.: So finding Janet was really a turning point for you.

Bill: Totally different. Totally. Totally different world. And as much as uh everybody coexisted, you know uh, right now I don't know where half of my brothers are, and that kinda thing. So it, it's been the, the separation over the years. That goes back to when you're, when you're young, you know.

Dr. C.: Yeah. It feels like we are scratching on the surface of a lot of pain.

A comment such as this acknowledges Bill's prior pain, further enhancing the therapeutic empathic connection. While other psychotherapeutic approaches might explore the origins of this pain and its various consequences, Dignity Therapy gives patients permission to include only those memories and recollections that they wish to share with others. This is not to say that a psychotherapist might not revisit these issues at a later time, but doing so is not part of a Dignity Therapy agenda.

> **Bill:** Yeah. And uh, it's, it's unfortunate that, that has ruled my life, in many respects.
>
> **Dr. C.:** Hm.
>
> **Bill:** The, that, uh it took me, a long time to get over that, over [ ]. It's like when you're brought up in an environment and this, the, the, some things stick to ya and it's hard to get rid of it.
>
> **Dr. C.:** Um-hum.
>
> **Bill:** And it took, took me a long time and uh, it took the, you know, it took a, any kinda toll on my, any kind of relationships you know that.
>
> **Dr. C.:** Up until your marriage, or did it continue to contaminate others?
>
> **Bill:** Continued. Continued. Yeah. I had to get over a lot of different things. I had to first realize them first that I couldn't get over them. They dictated my life.
>
> **Dr. C.:** Bill, today needs to be about you. I sense that those memories and details are painful to look at. But are you able to say what Janet and your marriage helped you to achieve?

This comment allows the therapist to once again touch on Bill's pain (and not be dismissive of it), while turning back to the generativity agenda and Bill's thoughts about Janet and their marriage.

> **Bill:** I think the one major thing, ih, in, in ih with the marriage and with the children and everything else is, um, uh I started to learn how to love. And I think that was, a major realization for me that I didn't even know, I lacked, you know. It's easy to say I love you, um it's another to live with it.
>
> **Dr. C.:** Yes.
>
> **Bill:** And I think that's the biggest thing of it.
>
> **Dr. C.:** And you began to learn by connecting with your wife and shortly thereafter, children came on the scene, beginning with Donna.

By introducing the children, the therapist is attempting to chronologically move the interview forward, while at the same time being mindful of important material related to the generativity agenda.

> **Bill:** Um-hum. Bang-o yep.

Dr. C.: Why don't you share some of those memories with me, memories of fatherhood and being a young husband, and what it was like learning how to love.

Bill: Well ih, ih, children don't really look at you in the respect that they're seeing your faults. They see you as a, as the Daddy as the, the uh, savior type of thing of the, the, the, which, is not entirely true, but I mean they look at you, up to you, in a different light. So they don't care about your problems. It's what you've kind of giving them um on an honesty basis cause all they can be is honest.

Dr. C.: Yes.

Bill: Up to a certain age. And uh but they uh, um they just, they just don't, they don't play games, when they're little.

Dr. C.: Yes.

Bill: They're just open and honest and, yeah you can't help but embrace them and that's where the, the love part comes in. I mean you'd go through a wall for your, for your children. I mean there's no question about that.

Dr. C.: Yeah. . . . share a picture with me.

Bill: Um-hum.

Dr. C.: Take me back to some of those memories that must be flooding back; you know, as a young husband, discovering new feelings, children in your life. Take me back to a picture or two.

Bill: Getting our first house.

Dr. C.: What do you see? Where are you? Who's in the photograph?

Bill: Um. (slight chuckle) The first one is, the two of us scratching our head.

Dr. C.: You and Janet.

Bill: Yeah.

Dr. C.: OK. The two of you scratching your heads.

Bill: Yeah because, wow, we're gonna buy a house. It's gonna cost $13,000.00. Ah um, wow. How to work that out how we're going to scrape up the money for it. But we did. Yeah um.

Dr. C.: I take it your accounting skills helped. (slight chuckle)

Bill: Well, maybe (slight chuckle)

Dr. C.: (slight chuckle)

Bill: But it was uh, uh, um, buying the, a, buying the first house and, and again, uh I you know, may sound silly, but some of the best times we had in that house were the best parties we had. We'd invite the families and everybody over. We had some wild theme parties yeah. Um.

Dr. C.: Let's hear about your wildest.

Bill: We had a um, what did we call it. We called it a, a, uh, a July Christmas party held in January. And everybody had to come in the middle of winter.

Dr. C.: Right.

Bill: Dressed in um, their uh, uh summer attire. And they had, we, we um, got a Barbie pool, kids Barbie pool. We set that up in the a, in the rec-room, we put gold fish in it. We had mosquitoes and bugs and flies hanging around, and uh, everybody had to come with a lawn chair, and they all came and took over the house and that's, that was one of the best parties we ever had.

Dr. C.: Were the children around?

Bill: Oh yeah. Everybody. The families. All the families. All Janet's family and my, my uh, my brothers at that time uh came over. Everybody.

Dr. C.: And how about the kids, are they all on the scene? Who would have been born, and what ages would they have been?

Bill: Our children and um Janet's brothers and sisters um, um, they're the same age, within months of each other.

Dr. C.: Right.

Bill: So they all chummed around.

Dr. C.: All the cousins.

Bill: All the cousins and uh, uh you know the nephews and you know my, my uh, my children were called uncles to this, and you know there's two months difference between some of them. So that, that's the kind of family that was developed.

Dr. C.: Right. So when you think about that party, Donna, who is now 45 would have been. . . .

Bill: She would have been um, well probably about, ten.

Dr. C.: OK.

Bill: Yeah.

Dr. C.: So Ed would have been around seven and a, and David around five.

Bill: Yeah.

Dr. C.: This is just so I can get a picture of who was on the scene at that time.

Bill: Yeah. Yeah. They were, they were uh, uh we just uh, we entertained a lot and loved to entertain and Janet became a, excellent cook, like her mother.

Dr. C.: Right.

Bill: And um it was just, and that's the, the kind of thing that when, when events happened it was the family that got together. All the families. Hm. Except for mine.

Dr. C.: I was going to say that in some ways, it seems so ironic, because you came from a place that didn't have much in the way of happy family connection.

Bill: Hm.

Dr. C.: And yet, most of your adult life was spent in this wonderful environment of loving family and family connections.

Bill: Yeah and that's, that's why I say that's where I discovered what love was all about. Hm.

Dr. C.: So, as you talk about love and think about moving forward through your photograph album, where does you mind take you to next? What other memories come to mind, or other things would you like to share?

Bill: Um apart from, from just living I mean things didn't uh, it was just a matter of all being together with the family and that was, that was a big part of it that's the big thing. After that of course was having uh, uh grandchildren, except for the teenage years. The, the kids when they go through their teenage years that's a, that's a, that's a minefield that you have to work through.

At this point, given his reticence to share too many detailed memories, the therapist has determined that Bill might have things to say about some of the more reflective and less biographical questions within the Dignity Therapy framework. Given that Bill has just mentioned having to "work through" the minefield of raising teenagers, this seemed an opportune time to ask him about things he has learned from life.

Dr. C.: Are there things that you learned through that period or things that you found out as you walked through the minefield that you think are worth putting into words?

Bill: I learned things, uh about myself that I didn't, I didn't know I had that kind of um, ability to reason. When you're, when you're dealing with teenagers, there's, it's very difficult to, to come to, it, it there's so many gray issues. It's not just a. It's very easy to say "don't do this" and "don't do that," but it, it doesn't apply if they go away outside of the family and do what they wanna do and um, my one son, he was a bit of a rebel.

Dr. C.: Hm.

Bill: But um, uh the one thing was that they never. My wife could cut him down to size very quickly. He was a big boy he used to have his uh. He was a very physical kind of guy, but uh, she still can cut him down to size. But with, with me it was more. I became, I didn't realize that I was becoming friends with my uh children.

Dr. C.: Hm.

Bill: You know.

Dr. C.: Can you say more about that?

Bill: Well I, I took fatherhood seriously and you, you, I've always had uh, I don't, I'm not a friend to my children, I'm a father. They can make as many friends as they want.

Dr. C.: Right.

Bill: But they will only have one father and um, the, I didn't, realize until later when they got older, and then they looked at me differently too.

Dr. C.: Um-hum.

Bill: That we were becoming friends over that period of time, and it was uh, well friendship is not something that's easy to say you grab a hold of them and say yes it's gonna be uh, we're gonna be friends. I mean uh, I have very few friends. Um but my children now are my friends.

Dr. C.: You said a moment ago that the role of being a father was something you took very seriously.

Bill: Um-hum.

Dr. C.: I assume it's a role that you feel proud of or you see as being very important in your life.

Bill: Well ih, uh, yeah because, coming from the environment that I, that I, I did come from, uh it was important for me to have the family that I was getting, not that I had. It was important for me.

Dr. C.: So how would you describe yourself as a father, or how do you think your children would describe you as a father?

Readers should recognize that this is moving on to questions pertaining to roles and the things that patients take pride in.

Bill: Um, I think they knew that I was a bit of a softy, and I think they knew that no matter what, I would be there for them, and I was. Uh it's not uh again it, see I, I really believe that the only thing you can give your children is love and discipline and, and uh, uh I gave them both. Uh all of that with um, with love.

Dr. C.: Yes. You sound like a man who feels few or no regrets on the issue of fatherhood. It seems to be an area where feel you got it right.

While this comment is not designed to necessarily move the dialogue forward, it once again shows that the therapist is listening carefully, understands Bill's core values, and appreciates his achievements within the realm of fatherhood.

Bill: It's probably one of the only things I did get right (slight chuckle) you know, and uh ih, not that it was, it wasn't easy, but, it's one of the things that, that I probably did get right because and I say that because of my relationship with them now.

Dr. C.: Yes.

Bill: Not um, you don't think of it when you're doing it. Um but when you look back on it, uh yeah there was some things I did that, wrong but, I did more right than wrong.

Dr. C.: While we are talking about fatherhood, earlier on you mentioned "grand-fatherhood."

The issue of "grandfatherhood" is raised in light of its likely importance to the generativity agenda.

Bill: Yeah.

Dr. C.: Could you skip ahead to that page of the album to tell me a bit about that experience. What has it been like?

Bill: It's been just an absolute, sharing of, ih, it's a, it's love on a different issue and it's on a different plane. You don't know what, what. I don't uh, I don't have to worry about disciplining them, and they know that. They, they've got me tied around their little finger and, and that's fine with me.

Dr. C.: (slight chuckle)

Bill: Yeah. And it's just being with them is so much fun. I don't have to worry about, disciplining them or your know bringing them up. I do in the, in the grandfatherly sorta way but I mean I don't have to worry, there's no pressure on me, and I just have fun with them.

Dr. C.: As you talk about them Bill, does your mind take you to a place where you can see yourself with them? Perhaps doing the kind of things with them that bring you the sort of joy that you are talking about now?

Bill: Well when we, when we used to do an awful lot of uh sort of weekends together during the summer time, and again the family would get together on different weekends and that's ih the joy again of having the all the family there, uh together. And to have the, the kids uh, uh it just, they give you a new energy.

Dr. C.: Yes.

Bill: You know. And, and it's unconditional love. More so than you know, even your own children. Hm. It's just a different level all together.

Dr. C.: Bill, not having come from a place where you could learn about these kinds of loving relationships, how did you think you learned to be the kind of father and grandfather that you are?

This type of comment, which invites patients to reflect on the origins of a particular trait or attribute, often works in Dignity Therapy, as it connects people with formative experiences (relationships, places, events) that have made them who they are.

Bill: Maybe because um I didn't have a role model in that sense, that I think I, I had to learn as you go along, you know there's nothing there that said you know, step 1, step 2, step 3.

Dr. C.: So you've been making it up all these years.

Bill: I've been making it up (slight chuckle) and uh, totally.

Dr. C.: Yes.

Bill: And uh, but that's uh, again a, a, a that's not a bad thing.

Dr. C.: No.

Bill: You know. So I think you look back upon my relationship with my parents and the relationship with that I have with my children, I think maybe there is more value, that I needed the value of being a parent. Maybe that, maybe that, because I didn't get it before. I. I, I probably at least wanted it now. Yeah.

Dr. C.: Bill, clearly being a father and grandfather have been important to you. Are there other roles in your life that you think have been important or that you value or feel proud of?

Bill: Hm. (long pause) Actually, I don't find anything else that is really um, sparkling in my life that, that has the same value, as, uh as the family and as my children, ih that there's, there's, um, there's nothing else that I really achieved that even comes close to them.

Dr. C.: Since we are talking about your family, it seems to me that the other important relationship worth looking at is your relationship with Janet.

Bill: Yes. But I had to learn to make that what it is. I had to uh. My particular background did not give me an element of trust that I could have with people and that, really affects communication. And that's always been um, certainly a problem with me.

Dr. C.: Hm.

Bill: You know.

Dr. C.: You were mentioning how the two of you have shaped one another. Where do you feel the two of you are at now?

Bill: Um. Comfort.

Dr. C.: Comfortable with each other.

Bill: Yeah. I think uh, um, that may sound rather sterile in a way but it's not. It's, it's um, I know when not to talk to her. And she knows when she has to talk to me.

Dr. C.: Yes.

Bill: Yeah. You know. So, so that's um, it's not, it's, it's not everything is perfect, but we've, we've, we've come to be comfortable with each other and to know each other.

Dr. C.: Bill, today you and I are doing Dignity Therapy. You have the opportunity to talk about things you want to talk about; perhaps to say things you feel need to be said. So getting back to Janet, do you have things that you feel still need to be said or perhaps you might want to say again?

This harkens back to an issue, raised in chapter 4, regarding "the time being now." While Bill suggests that there are things between him and Janet that are unspoken, implicit or only intuitively understood, the therapist reminds him that "this is the time" that he can choose a different path, and say the things he feels need to be said. Reminding him that this is a rare and fleeting opportunity is part of the role of the therapist.

Bill: I'm not sure how to answer that. Um, apart from you know, discovering love, um that's, in a, a, she has always been somebody to take care of me or whatever, you know. So she's always made that effort which I haven't always done. Keep things separate, you know, keep things back don't get too close.
Dr. C.: Hm.
Bill: That's what you go through life fighting. Don't get too close.
Dr. C.: Back to that issue of connection.
Bill: So it's a big step to go to love you know. But the uh, uh, and I've had to learn that it's alright to take that step you know.
Dr. C.: Yes.
Bill: To, to, to uh, to trust. Yeah.
Dr. C.: You were telling me a few days ago when we first met, that this illness of yours was serious; that you and your doctors are worried that time, whatever time there is, might be limited.
Bill: Um-hum.
Dr. C.: I'm coming back to this question about whether there are things that you still need to say. Look, none of us know how long we have, but if time is limited, are there things that you feel you need to take the time to put in to words?

This is perhaps as confrontative as a therapist might be in Dignity Therapy. Knowing that Bill has a realistic sense of his prognosis, and that he is naturally reticent to express his feelings, the therapist felt this admittedly confrontative approach was appropriate. As in any therapeutic situation, clinical intuition and judgment should be the final arbiter of when and how to proceed.

Bill: Just that um, love is somewhat precious to me and I don't always share it, uh, enough. I certainly do with my, my family but even that's not enough you know.

Love's a scary thing. You know to jump into and, and to be, to make that kind of commitment, to be spiritually connected. It's uh, it's a scary thing for me, always has been. Uh, but I've, I've, I think I've overcome an awful lot of that but I haven't. I will never totally get rid of that uh completely. You can make a complete commitment to your children. That's, that's no problem. The, I mean, you'd die for them, that's no problem. But to fall in love with somebody and to live with them and to uh, um want to, ih be with them despite their failings and my failings you know, that, that's a discovery. That's a long journey and I don't think it's over. So I can say I love my wife, and I love my children and uh, but ih tomorrow, it's another step.

Dr. C.: Is it frightening Bill, to think that the time to say all of the things that you find so difficult to say, may be running out?

Bill: That's a, totally. Uh time, I'm scared to death that I'm running out of time.

Dr. C.: So while there is still time, what do you want your wife to hear you say; what do you want your children to hear you say? Are you able to push aside some of that fear and say what you need to say?

Bill: I can say that I love them, but, but I say that anyway. And they say it back. So it's not in search of something that I haven't said to them before. I think the hardest, the, the thing is, to feel that I'm not gonna be with them.

Dr. C.: Hm.

Bill: That I'm not gonna be able to take care of them. That um, it, it's ih, I feel like I'm deserting them. Yeah. And that's um, that's something I can't, I can't deal with. I don't know how, I don't know how to deal with that. I don't. I, I, I, I want to, I want to protect them and I'm not gonna be able to do that, no matter what happens.

Dr. C.: One thing that you're doing today, I suppose to protect them or to help them, is to share your words. That's what you and I are doing. That's what this is about. This statement is meant to acknowledge Bill's pain, while reminding him that everything he is able to share within Dignity Therapy may protect, and provide comfort to, his family well into the future.

Bill: Hm.

Dr. C.: Bill, are there hopes, wishes, or dreams that you would want to share with them? Perhaps advice or direction you would hope to offer?

Bill: Oh. I look at my grandchildren and I think you know just don't sell yourself short. Go for it.

Dr. C.: You better explain to them what you mean by that. Just pretend that they're listening, because at some point they will be reading this.

Bill: They gotta live life true to themselves. That's, and that's it. They can't, they can't live it for everybody else and when I said don't sell yourself short, just go for it, with, what you got in here. You've all got personalities, you've, that, you've all got warmth, you all got compassion. You got, ih, they're all good people. You know. Just go with confidence that they are good people and, they don't have to sell themselves short to anybody. Be honorable be, be, uh, um, be honorable to, everybody else but be honorable to mostly to yourself, and within that, you'll discover your own love and your own um capacity for living. Uh and my, my children it would be, well.

Dr. C.: Are these words for all of your children or do you have specific words for each child?

Bill: Well each child, each um, each grandchild is a separate, boy they're totally different people. Uh, different personalities and they have a different um, outlook on life. I, I, I say I hope they can, can maintain the innocence that they've got now and carry that on ih, ih through life because, they hang on to that, that ih, it's, it's it um. If they can retain their personality and retain their, their honor.

Dr. C.: Um-hum.

Bill: They'll, they'll be ih, you can't, you can't look at each of them separately and say.

Dr. C.: Yeah.

Bill: You know, step 1, step 2, uh because uh, because they're different personalities. I mean Lindsay is one personality, ih la, she's a, she's um, she's a funny kid and I hope she can hang on to that and I hope that, you ih, ih tha, that, that doorway she's going through starting into that teenage, year, years that are, they're so tough for kids nowadays, but ih it's just all three of them I think it took.

Dr. C.: So you're referring to your eldest grandchild now?

Bill: My eldest grandchild Samantha, she's.

Dr. C.: Right.

Bill: She's just going into university or gone into university. She's on a, you know, on a different. She's facing life big time now and, just be true to the self, and you know that's what, what they can pay for, my, my.

Dr. C.: How bout Jack and little Cole?

Bill: Jack and little Cole well they're just so small.

Dr. C.: (slight chuckle)

Bill: That ih, it, it would be the same thing, and uh, if anything I could just hope they can keep smiling.

Dr. C.: Hm.

Bill: They're so funny, they're so full of life and laughter and they love laughing. I just hope they, they forever laugh. You know. Uh.

Dr. C.: And your own children, hopes, wishes, and dreams for each of them.

Bill: They've done so well that's, they've reached their own level already. They.

Dr. C.: You said earlier that you were worried about not being here for them. So I just wondered if you had some specific words for them?

Bill: Well again, we love each other so, its, um, I think if they'd, wouldn't take the world so seriously, let the world come to them, don't take the world so seriously. If they, they sometimes take the world on their shoulders and, I know I've been there. They don't have to.

Dr. C.: Hm

Bill: Just uh, um David is a funny guy, great personality. He gets along well with everybody, and, he's great at going out and getting people worked up and uh, for a project or whatever. And Donna runs her own business. She's a, she can be tough as nails sometimes but, she's just so vulnerable. Um, and again she doesn't have to take the world on if she'd just, lighten up.

Dr. C.: She'll, she'll know what you mean?

Bill: She'll know what I mean.

Dr. C.: (slight chuckle) And Ed.

Bill: And Ed. Here's a guy who loves his children so much and he's, he's so afraid sometimes. He, he's just starting to learn, how, his children love him.

Dr. C.: Hm.

Bill: And.

Dr. C.: It sounds like he reminds you of you.

Bill: Yeah. I think so. I think he, he's, he was so afraid of making a commitment, about getting married and then once he made it he wanted to be, the best at what he was doing and the thing was, he was the best he didn't have to. No. He. Get rid of your fears. He's had some fears, he's had some struggles, some.

Dr. C.: Hm.

Bill: There, there, there. I think his children are winning out.

Dr. C.: This could be a stretch, but I sense that you and Ed have walked a similar path. That being the case, are there lessons you've learned that you might want to pass along his way?

Bill: Oh, I've told him already. We've had uh, we've had some discussions.

Dr. C.: Right.

Bill: And, um, he uh, he just yeah. He's so willing ta take on the world that he doesn't have to.

Dr. C.: OK.

Bill: Yeah. And he is, he is learning a little bit to, to uh, ih not do that.

Dr. C.: And finally Bill, what about Janet? What are your hopes for her?

Bill: Well I hope she can have a party.

Dr. C.: (slight chuckle)

Bill: After I'm gone. Maybe a, uh, another Christmas. July Christmas in January party.

Dr. C.: Right.

Bill: And um, have everybody over and, and then I know, she's gonna be alright. She can take care of herself. She's gonna be, although um, she's taken care of me more than I've taken care of her, so she's, she's gonna be alright. Uh, you know. Uh I love her, and, she's just become a wonderful, woman. Hm.

Dr. C.: And in saying that she can take care of herself, do you have words that might help her accomplish that?

Bill: You know, ih, it's just that she knows I love her.

Dr. C.: Um-hum.

Bill: I know she loves me. I know she can take care of herself, and no matter what, I try to put on that, there's nothing, um, it's just after all these years, you know when, you are, I hate the thing of, we're just, together, you know.

Dr. C.: Um-hum.

Bill: We're bonded, you know. There's nothing else. I, ih, ih, I don't, I feel guilty about my mistakes that I've made, uh with her, but I know, she doesn't, she's, she, she doesn't hold them against me.

Dr. C.: Um.

Bill: And I, I don't hold anything against her. We've.

Dr. C.: All is forgiven.

Bill: All is forgiven, yeah. Oh, ten times more, all is forgiven. There is nothing to forgive.

Dr. C.: Any thoughts about what you hope might be in store for her?

Bill: Well, I think I'd be pissed off, but if, she's gonna meet a guy, get somebody who's rich and take her places, we never went to.

Dr. C.: Yeah.

Bill: But uh, uh, I hope she finds ih you know, life after. It's not. I don't want it to end for her. She's, she's got a life to live, but I want her to, to live that life. Life is for the living really.

Dr. C.: Yeah. Bill you must be getting a little wee bit tired. Uh we've been at this for just about an hour. Um, how are you feeling?

There have been many times, during the course of Dignity Therapy, that dying patients have given their partners explicit permission to find other life partners. As part of his Dignity Therapy, one gentleman said, "Our life together has been about happiness; I hope she understands that I would want her to find someone after I'm gone and for her to continue to be happy." While Bill is not quite as clear, in his own way, he is able to offer his wife this parting gift, a gift that may alleviate future feelings of guilt, as she tries to put together her life after Bill.

BILL'S GENERATIVITY DOCUMENT

Dr. Chochinov: Bill, can you tell me a bit about your life, particularly the things you remember most or would want your family to know?

Bill: Well I guess one does look back on their life when confronted with all of this. I'm not sure what kind of an exciting life I've led. I was around twenty when I went into accounting, and did accounting for a number of years. I later went into consulting with my own company. Accounting is not a very exciting career—it's pushing paper around. By the time I was twenty-four, I was a chartered accountant, *and* I got married. Finding a vocation and getting married wasn't something we planned. It just happens. When you're young there's not much thought of the future. It's just what you're doing now.

Several segments of dialogue were combined within the preceding paragraph, that is, "Accounting is not a very exciting career. It's pushing papers around" appears later in the original conversation but was moved, in order to achieve a more streamlined, chronologically coherent document.

Getting married was the most important thing that happened to me at that stage of my life. The next most important thing, that had any kind of meaning, would have been having children. I sort of lucked out with Janet, my wife, because she went along with my particular dreams and chasing things. Janet and I belonged to the same church—that's where we met. Through different socials at the church, we started to go around together. The first time I went out with her, I invited Janet *and* another girl to a party at the same time. That was exciting, but it ended up the other girl didn't take too kindly to it!

I remember trying to neck with Janet. That was a big thing for me. I wasn't nervous or frightened, not at that stage. I just wanted to neck! I had to think whether to take that to another step. I would drive her home, and we'd park outside of her house. Of course we'd do some necking there, until her mother would flip the *light* switch on! That meant it was time to come in. We've been married for forty-five years now.

The word "light" has been added to "switch" for clarity. The last sentence has been taken from the framing discussion with the therapist.

Interviewer: What was it about Janet that made you feel you had "lucked out?"
Bill: I guess it was finding somebody that I never had in my life, finding somebody that was missing. I didn't know that at the time. I didn't analyze it that way. Really it was just the total attraction. Looking back on it, I didn't know there was something missing in my life, but she certainly filled that void.

The sentence, "Um. You know the, it wasn't uh something that clicked and that turned around and said you know" was not included, as it added nothing by way of clarity or content.

We were going around and all of a sudden it was like, "Well, lets get married." We talked about children and things like that, but it wasn't like a light bulb went on. It's been something that we grew together, and it's been that way ever since. Not that she hasn't wanted to kick my ass once in a while! I don't understand people when then say *love at first sight*. It certainly wasn't with me, but it's like I've never been without her. We're opposites. Because of her personality she wants to be very organized and take care of things. But her personality is also one of laughter. I remember her whole family was the same way. She was the oldest of eight children, and they lived in a small house that was a joy to go to. It was always fun. She brought that joy and her mother's cooking to our marriage.

The participant used the word "basically" several time. Similar to the phase "you know," this can interrupt the flow of the narrative but, on the other hand, may be part of the participant's communication style. The therapist needs to decide, during the editing, when to include these words, to maintain the patient's unique voicing, and when, for the sake of clarity and flow, to delete them.

The participant's sentence, "Her, her personality apart from being very, wanting to be very organized and taking care of things and, and that kind of thing" does not read well in the narrative. This is an example of the importance of "cleaning up" the transcript and ensuring it flows well. In the final version, the wording is, "Because of her personality she wants to be very organized and take care of things."

Her family was such a different family than mine. When I think about that time, I think about being in the kitchen. Everybody gathered there. It didn't matter what the occasion. At every occasion, everybody ended up in the kitchen. That large family, standing around a kitchen, and laughing, that's what I remember. I remember we always used to go over there for Sunday dinner. Again it was everybody crammed in that kitchen, laughing and having a good time. We would laugh about anything and everything. Janet's mother died of cancer, and I said at the funeral, "I always remember the house with laughter." I still do. The house is still there and her dad still lives in the house. There were lots of beautiful memories in that house.

The previous paragraph is a distillation of two pages of original dialogue.

Dr. C.: Are there earlier memories that you might wish to talk about?

Bill: My upbringing wasn't the happiest of upbringings, so the memories that I have of that time are short. I don't really dwell on those times. I was the youngest of five boys. I remember things like the old car, a Model T Ford. I was just I kid, ten or twelve years old, when my brothers went together and bought the car. We used to have a field next to our house, and they would park the car out in the field and stand around like a bunch of peacocks, strutting their stuff, because they had a car! I can see my big brothers, standing there. My brother's got the car now.

We used to play ball and that kind of thing in the field. I remember my dog Skippy, a Cocker Spaniel. I don't even think that dog was really ours. It was our neighbor's, but we inherited it. We stole it! I had another dog, Prince, a cross between an Irish Setter and Black Lab. He was my pal. After we got married, they had to put Prince down. That was the end of an era for me and the beginning of a new one.

I came from a totally dysfunctional family in many respects and not a very happy one. I guess wanting to get married was part of my escape from that. I was twenty-four at the time and still living at home, even though I didn't like living at home. Finding Janet gave me a totally different world. As much as everybody coexisted, right now I don't know where half my brothers are. It's been a separation that goes back to when we were young. It's unfortunate that my early family life has ruled my life in many respects. It took me a long time to get over that. When you're brought up in an environment, some things stick to you and are hard to get rid of. It took a toll on any kind of relationships I've had, and it's continued to take a toll. I had to get over a lot of different things. I had to first realize that I couldn't get over them. They dictated my life. I think the one major thing with the marriage and the children is that I started to learn how to love. I think that was a major realization for me that I lacked knowing how to love. It's easy to say, "I love you," but it's another to live with it. I think that's the biggest thing.

For example, children don't really look at you in the sense that they're seeing your faults. They see you as the daddy, as the savior, which is not entirely true, but they look up to you in a different light. They don't care about your problems. You're telling them things on an honesty basis because all they can be is honest, up to a certain age. And they don't play games when they're little. They're just open and honest. You can't help but embrace them, and that's where the love part comes in. I mean you'd go through a wall for your children. There's no question about that.

Dr. C.: Are there some pictures from that time that are coming to your mind?

Bill: Getting our first house. The first picture I see is of Janet and I scratching our head, because we thought, "We're going to buy a house. It's going to cost $13,000.00. Wow! How are we going to scrape up the money for it?" But we did. Some of the best times we had in that house were the parties we had. We'd invite all Janet's brothers and sisters, my brothers and all the children. They would take over the house. Our children were all around the same age, within months of each other, so they all chummed together. We had some wild theme parties. One of them we called "a July Christmas Party Held in January." Everybody had to come in the middle of winter, dressed in their summer attire, with a lawn chair. We got a kid's Barbie pool, set it up in the rec-room and put gold fish in it. We had mosquitoes, bugs and flies hanging around too. That was one of the best parties we ever had.

That's the kind of family that developed. We entertained a lot and loved to entertain. Janet became an excellent cook, like her mother. When any event happened, the family got together. That's why I say that's where I discovered what love was all about. The family used to get together on different weekends during the summer. Again it was the joy of having the all the family together. Apart from living, it was a matter of all being together with the family.

Dr. C.: Are there things that you learned through that period?

Bill: I learned things about myself. I didn't know I had that ability to reason. When you're dealing with teenagers, there are so many gray issues. It's very easy to say, "Don't do this and don't do that," but it doesn't apply if they go outside the family and do what they want to do. When the kids went through their teenage years—that was a minefield you had to work through. My one son was a bit of a rebel and a very physical kind of guy, but my wife could cut him down to size very quickly. She still can cut him down to size.

Being a father has been very important to me, because coming from the environment I did, it was important for me to have the family that I was *getting*, not that I had. I think the kids knew that I was a bit of a softy, and I think they knew that no matter what, I would be there for them. I really believe that the only thing you can give your children is love and discipline, and I gave them both. Fatherhood is probably one of the only things I did get right, and it wasn't easy. I say that because of my relationship with them now. You don't think of it when you're going through it, but when you look back on it, you see there were some things I did wrong, but I did more right than wrong.

The word "getting" is italicized in order to give it appropriate emphasis.

I didn't realize that I was becoming friends with my children. I took fatherhood seriously, and I wasn't a friend to my children. I'm a father. They can make as many friends as they want, but they will only have one father. I didn't realize until later, when they got older, that they looked at me differently too. Friendship is not something where you grab a hold of people and say, "Yes we're going to be friends." I have very few friends, but my children now are my friends.

Being a grandfather has been love on a different plane. In that part of your life you go into a different stratosphere. I don't have to worry about disciplining them or bringing them up, and they know it. I do it in the grandfatherly sort of way, but there's no pressure on me, and I just get to have fun with them. They have me tied around their little finger, and that's fine with me. Being with them is so much fun. The grandkids give you a new energy and unconditional love – more so than your own children. It's a different level altogether. I didn't have a role model in that sense, and I had to learn as I went along. There's nothing that said, "Step 1, step 2, step 3." I've been making it up totally, but that's not a bad thing. (When I look back on my relationship with my parents and the relationship that I have with my children, I think that I needed the value of being a parent. Maybe because I didn't get it before, I at least wanted it now.)

The last two sentences seem somewhat vague; they would require clarification from Bill in order to remain within the final document.

Dr. C.: Are there other roles in life that you take pride in?

Bill: Actually, I don't find anything else sparkling in my life that has the same value as the family and my children. There's nothing else that I really achieved that even comes close to them. I had to learn to make marriage what it is. My particular background did not give me an element of trust that I could have with people, and that really effects communication. That's always been a problem with me.

The interviewer asked a question in between the participant's second sentence and third. " . . . the other important role and the other important relationship here is the relationship with Janet." In order to keep the flow of the narrative and ensure clarity, the therapist took the original words, "But I had to learn to do that too," and revised them to, "I had to learn to make marriage what it is." This does not change the meaning, but certainly brings clarity, while eliminating the therapist's unnecessary words.

> Right now, Janet and I are comfortable with each other. That may sound rather sterile, but it's not. I know when not to talk to her, and she knows when she *has* to talk to me. Not everything is perfect, but we've come to be comfortable with each other and to know each other.

Again to ensure clarity, the words of the therapist have been added to the participant's. The therapist asked, "Where do you feel that the two of you are at now?" and the participant answered, "Comfort." The therapist responds, "Cause you're comfortable with each other?" and the participant responds, "Yeah." The resulting sentence segment reads, " . . . we've come to be comfortable with each other. . . ."

> Dr. C.: Are there things you would like a chance to say or say again to Janet?
>
> Bill: I'm not sure how to answer that. Apart from helping me to discover love, she has always been somebody to take care of me. She's always made that effort, which I haven't always done. I am one to keep things separate, keep things back and not get too close. That's what you go through life fighting. "Don't get too close." It's a big step to go to love, but I've had to learn that it's all right to take that step—to trust.
>
> Love is somewhat precious to me, and I don't always share it enough. I certainly do with my family, but even that's not enough. Love's a scary thing to jump into, to make that kind of commitment and to be spiritually connected. It's a scary thing for me, always has been, but I think I've overcome an awful lot of that. I will never totally get rid of that. You can make a complete commitment to your children. That's no problem. You'd die for them. But to fall in love with somebody and to live with them and to want to be with them, despite their failings, that's a discovery. That's a long journey, and I don't think it's over. I can say I love my wife, and I love my children, but tomorrow, it's another step. I'm scared to death that I'm running out of time.
>
> Dr. C.: Are there things you would want to say to your children?
>
> Bill: I can say that I love them, but I say that anyway, and they say it back. So it's not in search of something I haven't said to them before. I think the hardest

thing is to feel that I'm not going to be with them. I'm not going to be able to take care of them. I feel like I'm deserting them, and that's something I can't deal with. I don't know how to deal with that. I want to protect them, and I'm not going to be able to do that, no matter what happens.

The word 'gonna' was changed to "going to"—again word revisions are an important consideration/undertaking for the therapist. Using the colloquialism in this instance felt like it might detract from this profoundly poignant moment.

Dr. C.: Are there wishes you have for your grandchildren?

Bill: I look at my grandchildren and think, "Don't sell yourself short. Go for it with what you've got in here—your heart." They have to live life true to themselves. That's it. They can't live it for everybody else. They've all got personalities, they've all got warmth, and they've all got compassion. They're all good people. Just go with confidence that they are good people and don't have to sell themselves short to anybody. Be honorable to everybody else, but be honorable mostly to themselves, and within that they'll discover their own love and their own capacity for living.

For the sake of clarity, the words "your heart" have been added to the second sentence; when he spoke these words, he made the gesture of holding his hand over his heart.

Throughout the original document, the participant uses the second person, "you," and the third person, "they," in reference to his family. To be consistent, the edited document refers to the family in the third person, "they."

You can't look at each of them and say, "Step 1, step 2," because they're different personalities. Lindsay is one personality. She's a funny kid, and I hope she can hang on to that through the teenage years that are just starting for her. It's so tough for kids nowadays. Dorie. . . . . *

My eldest grandchild Samantha has just started university. She's facing life big time now, and I hope she can be true to the self. Jack and little Cole, well they're just so small, but it would be the same thing for them. I hope they can keep smiling. They're so funny, so full of life and laughter, and they love laughing. I just hope they forever laugh.

---

* Dodie's name was mentioned in the framing conversation, but there was no mention made of her in this portion of the transcript. The therapist should bring this

to the participant's attention and ask what he would like to add about Dorie. Names, accuracy in spelling, and fairness in the attention paid to individuals can be important for those receiving the transcript.

Dr. C.: What are your hopes and wishes for your children?

Bill: They've done so well. They've reached their own level already. We love each other. I would tell them to let the world come to them and don't take the world so seriously. They sometimes take the world on their shoulders. I know; I've been there. They don't have to. Donna, our oldest is 45 and runs her own business. She can be tough as nails sometimes, but she's just so vulnerable. And again, she doesn't have to take on the world. If she could just lighten up; she'll know what I mean. Ed is forty-two years. Here's a guy who loves his children so much, and he's so afraid sometimes. He's just starting to learn how his children love him. I think he was so afraid of making a commitment, like getting married. Then once he made it, he wanted to be the best at what he was doing. The thing was, he was the best, and he didn't have to try. He's had some fears, some struggles, but I think his children are winning out. I would tell him to get rid of his fears. I've told him these things already. We've had some discussions. He's so willing to take on the world, and he doesn't have to. He is learning not do that. David is forty and a funny guy, great personality. He gets along well with everybody, and he's great at going out and getting people worked up for a project.

Each child, each grandchild is a totally different person, with different personalities and a different outlook on life. I hope they can maintain the innocence they've got now and carry that on through life. I hope they can retain their personality and their honor.

Dr. C.: What are your wishes for Janet?

Bill: Well I hope she can have everybody over for a party after I'm gone. Maybe another *July Christmas in January party*. I know she's going to be alright. She can take care of herself. She's taken care of me more than I've taken care of her, so she's going to be alright. She's become a wonderful person. I love her and I know she loves me. We're bonded. There's nothing else. I feel guilty about mistakes that I've made with her, but I know she doesn't hold them against me. I don't hold anything against her. All is forgiven. There is nothing to forgive.

I think I'd be pissed off, but if she's going to meet a guy, get somebody who's rich, who can take her places we never went to. I hope she finds life after. I don't want it to end for her. She's got a life to live, and I want her to live that life. Life is for the living really.

During the course of his debriefing, Bill—still in character—had the following reflections to share on his experience.

Finishing this, I am feeling somewhat subdued and maybe even content. I guess one needs to stop and look back over their life at a particular time. I think when you're in a health crisis situation you're forced to do that. I didn't know where this journey was going to take us. I'm surprised where we went. There are places that we haven't gone and we wouldn't go. The worst part I've had to deal with is something that I've put back—my upbringing. When I look at it, it helps me to understand who I am, but it doesn't solve any of the problems that I've had or that have lingered on. I think that story is going to need some dynamite. I think the biggest fear is going there, and not knowing what you're going to find out. But my family is the most important thing and that's the thing that we talked about the most.

As is made clear in the previous two examples, the verbatim transcripts provide the raw material for what the editor then turns into a pristine narrative, which we call the *generativity document*. Obviously, different editors will make different decisions in determining how to shape the document to the best of their abilities. However, so long as the basic principles of editing are adhered to, as outlined in chapter 5, the story and the essence of the message that the patient has to convey should remain unchanged. What does happen over time, with practice and experience, is that the transitions between various facets of the patient's responses are made smoother, and the process itself feels less daunting.

It is also worth noting just how different the original and the edited documents read, one from the other. The stories and overall content that the original and final edited document has to convey are identical, and yet, the experience of reading them is profoundly different. In general, the difference between the original and final document intensifies, as the patient, and his or her ability to respond to questions with spontaneity, energy and depth, diminish in the face of deteriorating health. So long as the editor remains committed to the therapeutic contract, that is, helping patients convey all they wish to within their Dignity Therapy, editing will remain a substantive element of providing them an all important, helping hand.

7

MOVING FORWARD

I know a little bit, about a lot of things, but I don't know enough about you.
—Peggy Lee, 1946

Dignity Therapy, in and of itself, is a story that continues to unfold. Colleagues from far and wide keep me apprised of how they are using it. Some contact me for advice regarding how to incorporate it into research initiatives, while others write to let me know they have been using it regularly since hearing me speak or having attended one of my workshops. For instance, a colleague from New Zealand, Dr. Peter Huggard (Faculty of Medicine and Health Science, Auckland) was recently in touch, letting me know that since my visit almost five years ago, dignity-conserving care has been incorporated into their graduate course in therapeutic communication and in other teaching with health professionals. A team of biographers working at Mercy Hospice in Auckland has adopted the questioning structure of Dignity Therapy in their work with patients near the end of their life as they write their personal stories; and for whom a full, multiple interview life story process is not possible. For the past two years, San Diego Hospice has employed Dr. Lori Montross as a full time Dignity Therapist.

Another colleague, Yasunaga Komori, whom I met the last time I was last in Japan, invited me to coauthor a case book with him, based on his clinical experiences of doing Dignity Therapy with patients nearing end of life. This book was recently published in Japan; a Korean translation has also just come out.[1, 2] Other colleagues in Denmark and Quebec have had regular contact over the last few years, advising me about their Dignity Therapy research and the progress they have made. In both instances, results have now been published and provide further evidence of Dignity Therapy's efficacy.[3,4] Another publication, providing an overview of Dignity

Therapy, has appeared in a book entitled *IPOS* (International Psycho-Oncology Society) *Handbook of Psychotherapy in Cancer Care.*[5] This rapid dissemination begs some important questions; questions that ought to be considered as clinicians and researchers in various settings anticipate how to move Dignity Therapy forward.

IS THERE CURRENTLY SUFFICIENT EVIDENCE TO SUPPORT THE APPLICATION OF DIGNITY THERAPY?

As previously indicated, the evidence in support of Dignity Therapy continues to mount. Study after study indicates that patients like and feel satisfied with it, and report that it heightens their sense of dignity, meaning, and purpose; spiritual well being and quality of life. Furthermore, there is evidence showing that family members feel it offers benefits, both it terms of how they perceive it helped their now deceased loved one and the comfort it provides during their time of grieving.

Colleagues in Copenhagen, including Lise Jul Houmann, Morten Aagaard Petersen, and Mogens Groenvold published a Dignity Therapy study. Like our own phase I trial, they discovered that most patients nearing end of life found it helpful and believed that it helped their relatives.[3] They also reported that it seemed to heighten patients' sense of purpose, dignity, and will to live. This particular study also included a follow-up evaluation, one month after returning the document. While patients' health had deteriorated over this time interval, some parameters of existential well-being—including sense of dignity and meaning—showed improvement.[3]

Another trial of Dignity Therapy, done in Quebec City with a cohort of French speaking palliative care patients, was recently published.[4] This study, carried out by Dr. Pierre Gagnon and others, reported additional strong support for Dignity Therapy as an end-of-life intervention. The majority of patients found that Dignity Therapy was helpful and heightened their sense of meaning, purpose, and overall sense of dignity. Of note, this particular study also revealed evidence regarding Dignity Therapy's potency as a bereavement intervention. The majority of families felt that it had been an important component of their deceased loved one's palliative care, and most would recommend it to other patients and families facing end-of-life circumstances. One family member had the following to say: "Without it [Dignity Therapy] I think I would not have passed through [the grief]. It helped me enormously."

However, amid these favorable results, there is a need to strike a cautionary note. All of the studies thus far, including our own,[6] have provided Dignity Therapy to general palliative care populations. No study has yet attempted to use Dignity

Therapy exclusively in the context of marked distress. Although studies to date have shown almost universal satisfaction and an enhancement of end of life experience, what can we say about patients who are markedly distressed, or perhaps even clinically depressed? In those instances, is Dignity Therapy an appropriate and proven intervention? At this time, until further data is amassed, I believe the answer is no. This is not to say that it might not be used in conjunction with other standardized approaches. However, offering Dignity Therapy in lieu of conventional treatment for depression would be moving practice beyond the current evidence. What about patients who are requesting assisted suicide or euthanasia? Given that these patients often experience as sense of loss of meaning and purpose, this would be an intriguing population to Dignity Therapy to however, its efficacy in those circumstances has yet to be established. No doubt, future clinical trials will clarify the various opportunities and limitations of this novel psychotherapeutic approach.

HOW DO I BECOME SKILLED ENOUGH TO IMPLEMENT AND IMPROVE MY ABILITIES TO DELIVER DIGNITY THERAPY?

Like any new psychotherapy, no one book or single training seminar can make you fully competent. New skills and approaches take time to learn and incorporate into practice, and even more time to gain a sense of mastery. Those of us who have been doing Dignity Therapy for many years have come to realize that experience is a wonderful teacher. With humility as our ever-present co-therapist, we continue to learn from our patients and remain in awe of the things they manage to say and accomplish by way of Dignity Therapy.

As with all psychotherapies, some form of supervision is a wonderful way to improve skills and reflect on the quality and efficacy of one's work. Finding someone with more experience than you might be difficult, given that Dignity Therapy is still quite new on the palliative care scene. But there are ways of accelerating your learning. First, you might want to consider attending a Dignity Therapy Workshop. Our research group now offers annual intense Dignity Therapy training workshops in Winnipeg, Canada. It is too early to say how often these will be held, and much will depend on what demand there is for training. Readers considering this option may want to check www.dignityincare.ca, where updated training opportunities will be posted regularly. Peer-to-peer support is also a helpful way of learning. It provides a rich opportunity to see how others are carrying out this work, just as they, in turn, might be informed by how your practice of Dignity Therapy is taking shape.

One distinct advantage Dignity Therapy offers by way of skill enhancement is that the sessions are recorded. This means that there is a very clear record of how you are delivering Dignity Therapy. Also, so long as you are using tracking throughout the editing process, there is a very accurate paper trail for how you are progressing as a Dignity Therapy editor. Again, these documents offer the potential for Dignity Therapy education. All three versions of the transcripts (unedited, tracked edited, and final edited) can be shared with colleagues, either face-to-face or electronically. The latter raises the possibility of having international supervisory exchanges among those incorporating Dignity Therapy into their practice. Discussion boards, blogs, Facebook, all are ways of creating virtual communities with a vested interest in practicing, discussing, and becoming more adept at Dignity Therapy (readers can visit www.dignityincare.ca to learn about these training opportunities).

HOW MUCH DOES DIGNITY THERAPY COST AND HOW CAN RESOURCES TO SUPPORT IT BE FOUND?

Over the years, people have asked about the issue of cost. Most health care systems are stretched, with pressure of having to make do with less. No doubt, the idea of accruing further costs, for whatever purpose, may seem untenable. But before getting ahead of ourselves, let us look at the actual costs of Dignity Therapy. Programs or institutions already providing psychosocial care will, in most circumstances, cover the therapist's time. This time breaks down as follows; about one-half hour of the therapist's time to explain the intervention, answer questions, provide the patient with the Dignity Question Protocol, and arrange a follow-up time for the recorded interview; one hour for the actual taped Dignity Therapy session, with an extra half hour or so to set up and debrief; another half hour to one hour of face-to-face time with the patient is needed to review the edited document and take note of any changes that might be required.

If the therapist's time is covered within existing resources for psychosocial support, what are the additional or administrative costs for delivering Dignity Therapy? First, there is the cost of the transcription itself. This will of course vary, depending on how long patients speak and various factors that might influence the pace and clarity of their speech. We budget about C$200 per transcript. The other activity, which we feel is best done by the therapist, is editing. Like Dignity Therapy, editing is an acquired skill; you will get better at it and more efficient with practice. Nonetheless, one should set aside about double the time it took to conduct the interview itself. So as not to underestimate the resource implications, let us assume two to three hours are needed to edit a Dignity Therapy transcript. For argument sake, let us further assume that a therapist's time is billed at $100 per hour (this will vary, of course, depending on the disciplinary affiliation of therapists and the financial arrangements of their employment [e.g. fee for service, block funding, etc]).

This would bring the administrative cost of Dignity Therapy, including transcriptionist fees, to $400 to $500.

What are the challenges in finding the necessary resources to support Dignity Therapy? First, there is the not inconsiderable issue of overcoming a dominant bias that psychosocial interventions, even those that work, should cost nothing whatsoever. Consider for a moment how quickly a $500 challenge would be met, if we were discussing the release of a new pharmaceutical, shown to enhance sense of well-being, mood, and quality of life. If that were the case, such costs would be considered inconsequential. Relative to the cost of most palliative chemotherapy or radiation therapy, the cost of Dignity Therapy is, indeed, very inexpensive.

Bearing in mind the evidence supporting Dignity Therapy, there is a strong case to be made for its inclusion within state-of-the-art palliative care services. So long as programs are committed to being grounded in evidence-based approaches, they will need to identify a source for these very modest new funds. Some hospitals and institutions may absorb this cost; others may turn to health care or philanthropic foundations for support. Perhaps there may be a role for hospice organizations to help support the task of Dignity Therapy transcription by way of funding or the provision of capable volunteers. Whatever the model of funding, investing in an inexpensive and effective intervention that can provide comfort to patients and families and has the potential for multigenerational impact makes excellent common and fiscal sense.

WHAT IF FAMILY MEMBERS OR VOLUNTEERS WANT TO TAKE ON THIS WORK? IS THAT AN OPTION?

About a year ago, I had the good fortune of offering a Dignity Therapy Workshop in Sydney, Australia. Near the onset of the day, I was approached by an attendee who was very excited about the potential for Dignity Therapy to be administered by volunteers. While I did not have much time to respond to the idea, my tone must have given me away. Toward the end of the workshop, when we next managed to connect, she said, "I see why you were hesitant." And in truth, I am hesitant to suggest that Dignity Therapy is something that volunteers or family will be able to take on.

Without a doubt, families and volunteers play a profound role within the spectrum of end-of-life support. There are many elements of the Dignity Model that can inform how they might attend to the psychological, spiritual, and existential needs of someone whose illness is advancing toward death. From this model, we know that finding ways to value and affirm a patient's sense of personhood is a vital element of quality end-of-life care. Asking people questions about themselves, their past, what they care about—in fact, many of the questions within the Dignity Therapy protocol—are wonderful ways of sending the message that who they are, who they were, and what they still have to say is valuable. This value is conveyed in a very simple and tangible fashion by way of the listener being present, attentive, and appreciative of those disclosures that happen to be shared.

However, I see several obstacles in having volunteers and families administer Dignity Therapy. First is the simple fact that Dignity Therapy, like any other form of psychotherapy, requires a skill set that must be carefully and thoughtfully honed over time. People often assume that Dignity Therapy simply involves reading a list of questions (the Dignity Therapy question protocol) and passively recording the person's responses. If only it were so simple. Readers of this book should understand that while the questions provide a framework, the therapist must be highly skilled at eliciting responses, identifying important issues, engaging patients within the process; mitigating possible negative outcomes, and taking the patients' disclosures and weaving them into a cohesive and meaningful generativity document.

This is not to suggest that one must be a psychiatrist, psychologist, or trained psychotherapist to carry out Dignity Therapy. I have trained social workers and palliative care nurses to become very skilled Dignity Therapists. Family members have an added challenge that, in my opinion, would make doing Dignity Therapy with their loved ones particularly difficult. Anyone who has lost someone they love knows the intense, heart-wrenching feeling of watching a person close to them—perhaps someone whose life shaped and helped define their own—move toward death. This experience unleashes a cascade of feelings—anguish, pain, disorientation, grief—but one thing it does not bring is objectivity. To do Dignity Therapy, a degree of objectivity is important. Therapists need to be mindful of the overall process. They must be monitoring the clock, being sure that patients are able to complete the protocol within a timeframe that won't exceed the limits of their energy and current abilities. Therapists need to be monitoring whether patients are straying or moving away from a generativity agenda. Therapists must always be gentle but prepared to be directive, always in the service of helping patients achieve their Dignity Therapy goals.

While perhaps not obvious, the Dignity Therapist performs a skillful balancing act, which again, goes beyond what a family member could reasonably be expected to do. On the one hand, the therapist must provide affirmation in the here now; on the other hand, they must be mindful that there is a limited opportunity to have patients address various content that they wish to include in their generativity documents. A skillful therapist is able to achieve this balance, without ever sacrificing the quality of the therapeutic interaction. The ability to understand the psychology of why certain generativity messages might be difficult to reveal is also very helpful. These are often rooted in conflicted relationships or unresolved intrapersonal issues. For example:

A sixty-three-year-old gentleman disclosed early on in his interview that his parents were very emotionally reserved and undemonstrative in their affection toward their children and one another. This reticence to show feelings was a trait he, too, had acquired. Now, toward the end of his life, he was using Dignity Therapy to share memories, hopes, and dreams with his wife and two daughters. While he was able to provide stories and rich biography with little effort, his messages contained less in the way of emotional content toward his family. Noticing this, the therapist commented: "Peter, it seems like you've always had a hard time telling your family exactly how you felt about them. Do you think that today, given that this is your Dignity Therapy, you might be able to do this differently?" Offering this formulation, while gently delivered, was a rather provocative therapeutic maneuver. Nevertheless, in the hands of a skilled therapist, it can point toward openings and opportunities while leaving the patient in charge of how to proceed. In this instance, Peter was able to response, "I want them to know that I love them, I loved them, that I tried hard, and that I did my best."

CAN DIGNITY THERAPY BE DONE BY A THERAPIST WHO KNOWS THE PATIENT WELL?

This question actually came up at a recent Dignity Therapy workshop. Therapists attending this meeting asked if knowing the patient might create a different dynamic, compared to the patients our group has seen within the context of research. As researchers, we have no foreknowledge of who is being referred to our studies, nor do we have a prior, or any ongoing, clinical connection with the patient. So, compared to a patient being considered for Dignity Therapy within one's practice, the circumstances are quite different. The question, however, is whether those differences change the ability to undertake Dignity Therapy, and if so, how?

The most obvious difference is that the patient being enrolled from within someone's practice will be well known, or at least relatively well known, compared to the person doing this as part of a research study. Readers will recall that part of being a Dignity Therapist is "laying down dots," that is, providing patients with appropriate cues that allow them to more easily construct their responses to the question framework. Knowing the patient's history, in advance of actually doing Dignity Therapy, may offer the therapist some clear advantages. Recall that most patients use a portion of their Dignity Therapy to share stories or reminiscences that they feel are important or that they would want their families to know about. Knowing some of this information in advance of Dignity Therapy might ensure that therapists don't overlook these important recollections. Unlike researchers, who don't know what they don't know, the informed clinician can be mindful of significant oversights, so that carefully chosen dots can be provided in order to help direct patients toward meaningful disclosures. It is conceivable that knowledge is a double-edged sword. Perhaps, if the therapist knows the patient has had a difficult life, he or she may be disinclined to offer Dignity Therapy. This would be unfortunate, in that although our inclination might be to facilitate the telling of "good" stories, "sad" stories—stories of regret, betrayal, adversity, or conflict—can be equally important to tell, albeit more difficult to share.

Some therapists wonder whether knowing the patient, and knowing something of the patient's issues, will diminish from the poignancy of Dignity Therapy. In other words, if you already know something about the person, his or her core values and key messages, will the retelling of these feel redundant or even contrived? While time and experience will tell, my suspicion is that this will not be a significant problem. As therapists, while we have an awareness of the patients overall history, we tend to focus on areas of intra-psychic and interpersonal conflict. While some elements of Dignity Therapy will no doubt be drawn from those particular sources, it is extremely unlikely that they will be the exclusive domains of what informs Dignity Therapy.

There is also something about the idea of creating a permanent record that permeates the entire experience of Dignity Therapy. Knowing these conversations are recorded, and that they will serve as the basis of generativity documents, changes how patients approach sharing their stories, feelings, and thoughts. The spoken word is meant to convey meaning in the here and now, and is privy to only those within earshot. Recording the patient's words changes everything. Even if the therapist has previously heard some of these disclosures, facilitating permanence means transcending the here and now and creating the potential for a broad and even multigenerational audience. The idea that "your words may resonate across time, even beyond your death" makes the experience of doing Dignity Therapy both unique and profound.

Another question is whether therapists can undertake Dignity Therapy and somehow manage the tension between interpretive, uncovering methods and an approach whose primary ingredients are generativity and affirmation. Although separation between these would seem plausible, the real test comes when facing this in practice. Suppose for example that during the course of Dignity Therapy a patient reveals a major life trauma, for example, a history of being sexually abused. The correct therapeutic response, the only tenable therapeutic response, is to preempt Dignity Therapy and shift the focus of attention to this disclosure, guided by the patient's wishes and ability to do so. Acknowledging such profound trauma, but undauntedly trying to move forward with Dignity Therapy (or any other agenda, for that matter), could be experienced as an assault to the patient and a substantive violation of trust.

On the other hand, more subtle instances of having to choose between traditional therapeutic pursuits and Dignity Therapy are likely to be far more frequent. For instance, a Dignity Therapy patient recently disclosed, fairly early into his session, that he had had an unhappy childhood. The psychotherapist might be tempted to pursue this, by way of exploring the details of this unhappiness and how it influenced this man's psychosocial development. However, the Dignity Therapist, ever mindful of generativity and the need to provide affirmation, must sort out how to acknowledge and validate this disclosure while moving Dignity Therapy forward. A less experienced therapist might decide to avoid the issue entirely by inviting the patient to share memories arising exclusively after the gloom of childhood. While this might seem a reasonable way to pursue "good" stories, it also assumes that this direction is in accord with the patient's wishes. The approach the therapist used, to good effect in this instance, went as follows: "Doing Dignity Therapy should be about you and needs to be exactly what you want it to be. If you don't want us to visit your childhood, let's not. However, if there are episodes or memories from youth that you want, or feel are important, to be part of your Dignity Therapy, this would be the time for us to talk about them." At this point, the patient shared some poignant childhood memories, recalling how he had served as an apprentice to his father in a local community club.

ARE THERE STILL THINGS ABOUT DIGNITY THERAPY WORTH STUDYING? IF SO, HOW MIGHT RESEARCHERS TAKE UP THIS WORK?

While there have been several studies on Dignity Therapy, there is so much more to do and know. Among the most pressing questions are these: Who is Dignity Therapy most likely to benefit? What is the nature of the therapeutic effects wielded by Dignity Therapy? How can one measure the influence and benefits of Dignity Therapy?

Some clinicians are already beginning to apply Dignity Therapy more broadly than just end-stage cancer. This implies that the Dignity Model itself applies beyond cancer and possibly beyond just end-of-life care. Readers will recall that the themes and subthemes contained within the Dignity Model are quite universal, including influences on the body (Illness-Related Concerns), the social environment (the Social Dignity Inventory), and the psyche and spirit of patients nearing death (The Dignity-Conserving Repertoire). While this is not to say that the model can be applied indiscriminately, in terms of face validity it certainly would seem to resonate across a broad spectrum of the human experience. Our own research group has piloted Dignity Therapy in a cohort of frail elderly residents living in Personal Care Homes. This pilot was launched because of overlapping existential issues, which resonate in palliative care and the frail elderly. While the former are dying, the latter are moving closer toward the end of life. Although our findings (which will soon be reported within the peer review literature) suggest that there are differences in how Dignity Therapy operates amid the frail elderly, it does appear to be a viable and affirming intervention for this vulnerable population.[7]

We also have some experience using Dignity Therapy with patients who have amyotrophic lateral sclerosis (ALS). Although the ability to speak is often a substantive and rate-limiting factor, patience, creativity, and accommodation—such as using facilitated communication of some variety—can enable these patients to have a positive Dignity Therapy experience. In one instance, a gentleman with ALS who still had the manual dexterity to type was provided his Dignity Therapy transcript electronically. This allowed him to keyboard editorial changes and thus complete the document to his specifications. Colleagues in Australia, currently funded by the Motor Neurone Disease (MND) Association of Western Australia, are studying how Dignity Therapy might be applied in patients living with MND. And though many people have suggested that they see an application, or are in fact using Dignity Therapy in less acute palliative circumstances (for example, woman with Stage III or Stage IV breast cancer), I am not aware of any funded clinical trials examining its role in those specific patient populations.

One of the most substantive challenges facing researchers attempting to study Dignity Therapy is the whole issue of design and selection of outcome measures. Our recently completed randomized control trial used various approaches to discern differences across study arms.[5] However, showing significant changes across a broad spectrum of psychometric measures is difficult when examining patients with initial low base rates of distress. In other words, so long as protocols are reliant on demonstrating pre-intervention versus postintervention change on various dimensions of end-of-life experience, the ability to prove efficacy could depend upon how much initial distress a study cohort happens to contain. Invoking a medical comparison, demonstrating an agent's ability to mitigate fever or promote bone healing is highly dependent on the presence of fever or a broken bone, respectively.

There are instances, such as concurrent clinical depression, delirium, or an anxiety disorder, where indeed, something is *broken*, needing treatment and repair. Those complications lend themselves well to empirical inquiry, following conventional approaches that employ clinical trials, validated outcome measures, and standard statistical methods. There are challenges facing dying patients, however, which metaphorically, do not readily equate to something being *broken*. A heavy heart, a mournful soul, anguish in the face of loss—are these really complications along the pathway to death, or manifestations of our humanity and inescapable vulnerability? Rather than problems to be fixed or complications to be cured, perhaps our therapeutic responses need to embrace notions of witnessing, affirming and healing.

While these considerations may seem essentially philosophical, the implications for researchers are largely pragmatic. Some Dignity Therapy participants have said this process helped them achieve a sense of peace while nearing death; others have given spouses permission to find new life partners after they die. One patient sought her daughter's forgiveness for not having revealed the identity of her father until it was well too late. Another daughter told us that the only time her father ever indicated he loved her and was proud of her was in his Dignity Therapy document. These outcomes are hard to quantify, particularly within our armamentarium of psychometric measures. These results, nevertheless, are profound and real. Researchers examining Dignity Therapy should strive to capture this kind of data, although this may not be easily achieved within an exclusively quantitative paradigm. Qualitative approaches and measures that attempt to capture notions of self-worth, sense of peace or calm, dignity, meaning, spiritual well-being, or existential angst are all important protocol considerations.

WHAT ABOUT OTHER MODES OF GENERATIVITY?

By no means is Dignity Therapy meant to displace any other form of generativity that patients and families deem fitting. As in many things in life, what is important is how well matched the approach and the user of the approach happen to be. Creating video recordings, audio recordings; for patients so inclined, keeping a diary, or writing a series of letters for partners, children, and friends are all ways of trying to preserve the memory of someone about to die. Words are not the only mode of generativity. I recall an airline pilot dying of multiple myeloma; woodcarvings, rather than words, were his way of trying to leave a part of himself behind. Another patient approaching death discussed the various paintings she had produced, and which of her beloved family she thought each would most be suited to inherit. It is also worth noting that the need to focus on generativity will vary from one individual to the next. Some people may see their families, their life's work, and whatever mark they have made, big or small, as satisfying their generativity needs. The importance of and the need for a generativity outlet must be determined on a case-by-case basis.

WHAT ABOUT DYING CHILDREN? DOES DIGNITY THERAPY HAVE A ROLE TO PLAY?

While I have been asked this question many times, it is not one that I can answer from the perspective of experience. Our own research, and that of colleagues worldwide, has seen Dignity Therapy applied exclusively in patients, eighteen years of age or older. Given our bent to follow empirical leads, confining it to adults simply reflects that the Dignity Model itself is based on older patients with end-stage cancer. Hence, one cannot assume that the model applies well, beyond this specific demographic.

Our experience of Dignity Therapy thus far offers some clues as to whether it might have applications among younger dying patients. Existential insight and yearning for generativity are important motivations for most Dignity Therapy participants. Without these, Dignity Therapy does not usually resonate as a meaningful endeavor. Therefore, before determining an expanded role for Dignity Therapy, one must understand existential insight and generativity needs, and how these find expression in younger cohorts of dying patients. Like death awareness, these constructs are developmental in nature and evolve and mature with age. Future clinical work and careful study will determine whether Dignity Therapy has a role to play, and what protocol adjustments will be required to make it suitable and age appropriate (for example, using photographs, drawings, co-construction with parents; possible ancillary roles for siblings, and other close relatives and friends).

WHAT ABOUT THE ISSUE OF CULTURE AND DIGNITY THERAPY?

As previously indicated, Dignity Therapy has been introduced and/or studied in many countries around the world. Workshops have taken place in various centers across Canada and the United States. It has also been presented to audiences in China, Japan, Taiwan, Singapore; Australia, New Zealand, Israel; Cuba, Brazil, Argentina; and many centers throughout Europe (Switzerland, Portugal, Spain, Italy, Sweden, Austria, Scotland, England, Denmark, the Netherlands and Norway).

The experiences from two settings, where formal studies are currently under way, are worth noting with respect to cross-cultural considerations. Our colleagues in Denmark, who have been using and studying Dignity Therapy since 2003, have found it works well among Danish patients nearing end of life. However, they discovered that the idea of *taking pride in oneself* or one's accomplishments is not a good or comfortable cultural fit. For Danes, pride is akin to boastfulness or arrogance. Endorsing a sense of pride, given Danish sensibilities, is seen as crass and immodest. The implications for Dignity Therapy, however, are minimal. Subtle tweaking saw Danish therapists ask patients about their accomplishments, in terms of what they considered most important or meaningful, rather than framing this question in terms of personal pride.

Colleagues in Hong Kong, including Dr. Ceci Chan, Dr. Pamela Leung, Mr. Andy Ho, Dr. Rainbow Ho, and Dr. Xiaolu Wang, have pointed out another interesting cultural nuance with implications for Dignity Therapy. In the course of examining the Model of Dignity, these researchers at the University of Hong Kong have studied the Chinese notion of *face* and what this means in the context of nearing end of life. *Face* refers to how the Chinese are inclined to preserve their self-respect and self-identity. Conceptually, it is closely aligned with social relationships and network, along with the Eastern idea of collective autonomy. While they are still studying the model, this deeply held cultural outlook will no doubt manifest in some way—perhaps choice of content and the fashion in which loved ones will be addressed—within the course of undertaking Dignity Therapy.

Those interesting observations notwithstanding, Dignity Therapy seems to be easily and meaningfully applied across many different cultures. Readers should be mindful that the framework of questions is intended to be flexible and applied to the extent, and in a fashion, which patients find it guides them toward a satisfactory Dignity Therapy. Perhaps this is why protocol burden is never a problem, given that whatever the patient's circumstances, agenda, or cultural background, Dignity Therapy can be shaped based on exactly what the patient wants and needs it to be.

HOW SHOULD DIGNITY THERAPY BE EVALUATED?

The answer to this question largely depends on the context within which evaluation is being done. I have already addressed this question for those anticipating doing further research on Dignity Therapy. However, what about clinicians planning to introduce this into their practice? Although they are under no obligation to do so, it is advisable that some tracking method, which monitors how often Dignity Therapy is used, the circumstances of patient participants, and the responses of both the participant and family, be utilized. At a local level, this kind of paper trail could provide invaluable information for quality assurance purposes. Depending on the weight of the evidence, such documentation could also provide the justification for funding strategies to support Dignity Therapy.

Clinicians doing Dignity Therapy are invited to visit www.dignityincare.ca. It is only by gathering and sharing our collective experience that the field will move forward and help us gain further appreciation for the advantages and limitations of this novel and new therapeutic approach.

CLOSING THOUGHTS

Earlier on in this handbook, I promised to describe the first patient who completed Dignity Therapy. Ending in this way seems fitting, given that Dignity Therapy so readily evokes reminiscences spanning birth to death and the circle of life. It is time to close the circle on that particular gentleman's remarkable story.

When you first met him in chapter 1, he as identified as Mr. G., a sixty-eight-year-old married gentleman with an end-stage gastrointestinal malignancy. He had attempted to starve himself to death, given that his body was no longer cooperating with the many things he still yearned to do. Readers may recall, when I first met him for psychiatric consultation, he greeted me with the words, "If we were living in a certain European country, and I could press the button right now, I would!" Both of us knew exactly what button he was referring to.

Given that he was not suffering any particular psychiatric disorder that I could identify, I offered him Dignity Therapy. After carefully explaining the protocol (my first time having done so with an actual patient), he took a long pause before saying that this sounded "interesting" and he wanted to take part. Readers may also recall that before leaving him, and having made arrangements to return the following day to make the recording, I asked Mr. G. if he still wanted to "push the button now." His response indelibly shaped the next seven years of my program of palliative care research. "No," he said, " I'd like to do this first."

The following day I arrived to his room, mid-day, with tape recorder in hand. He was not having a particularly good day and indicated as much. He seemed more uncomfortable than the previous day and somehow less settled. I suggested that we could defer this session to another time, given that I wanted him to be in a good place to embark on this joint venture. While I began to make motions to leave, he caught sight of the tape recorder, and suggested that "we try." As soon as the audio recording begun, Mr. G. sat up in bed and for the next hour—gently guided by my questions—shared a lifetime of memories, spanning what had been a rich, complex, and very full life. He told the story of his birth family in Russia near the turn of the twentieth century, shared memories of his beloved, long deceased parents and the trauma of unforgettable violence and revolution. He went on to describe the arduous process of immigration to Canada, his marriage, and his experience of fatherhood and raising a family. Like most people, his life was one marked by both great tragedy and wonderful accomplishments. As he neared the completion of this Dignity Therapy, he offered individual blessings to each of his children, and expressed his love and wishes for his soon to be bereft wife.

Given the protocol we had established from the very outset of this work—and a necessary ethos of immediacy—we had his full interview transcribed and, within no more than two days, arrived back at his bedside with the finalized document. By this time, however, his condition had deteriorated further, and he was unable to provide any verbal response whatsoever. However, his wife, who knew about the study, happened to be with him, sitting at his bedside. As she took the generativity document from me, with tears in her eyes and a quiver in her voice, she said, "This will be a blessing for our family."

I have always considered looking after terminally ill patients and their families to be a privilege and a blessing. Prior to Dignity Therapy, it would have struck me as entirely unfathomable that a brief psychotherapeutic intervention might enhance a patient's sense of meaning, purpose, and dignity, offer comfort to the bereft, and have the potential for mutigenerational impact. And yet our research group and others abroad have shown Dignity Therapy capable of accomplishing those very things. The therapeutic doorways it has opened and the opportunities to provide comfort, mitigate suffering, and promote healing are unique and effective.

Although dying is inevitable, dying poorly ought not to be. In the tradition of the modern hospice movement, Dignity Therapy represents yet another way for clinicians to enhance the quality of life for patients nearing death. Dignity Therapy is by no means a panacea and not everyone will want or need this patient-affirming, meaning-enhancing approach. However, for patients and families so inclined, I have no doubt that you will be impressed and humbled by what Dignity Therapy might help them achieve. Your patients, their surviving loved ones, and perhaps generations to come will forever be grateful.

REFERENCES

1. Komori, Y & Chochinov, HM. Introduction to Dignity Therapy. Kongo Shuppan. 2011 (Japan)
2. Komori, Y & Chochinov, HM. Introduction to Dignity Therapy. Korea Hakjisa Publisher ISBN 978-89-6330-682-7. 2011.
3. Houmann LJ, Rydahl-Hansen S, Chochinov HM, Kristjanson LJ, Groenvold M. Testing the feasibility of the Dignity Therapy interview: adaptation for the Danish culture. BMC Palliat Care. 2010;9:21.
4. Gagnon P, Chochinov HM, Cochrane J, Le Moignan Moreau J, Fontaine R, Croteau L. *Psychothérapie de la Dignité* : Une Intervention pour Réduire la Détresse Psychologique Chez les Personnes en Soins Palliatifs. Psycho-Oncologie. 2010; 4:169-175.
5. Watson M, Kissane D, Handbook of Psychotherapy in Cancer Care. Wiley. 2011.
6. Chochinov HM, Kristjanson LJ, Breitbart W, McClement S, Hack TF, Hassard T, Harlos M. Effect of dignity therapy on distress and end-of-life experience in terminally ill patients: a randomised controlled trial. Lancet Oncol. 2011 August;12(8): 753–62
7. Chochinov HM, Cann B, Cullihall K, Kristjanson K, Harlos M, McClement SE, Hack T, Hassard H. Dignity Therapy: A Feasibility Study of Elders in Long-term Care. Journal of Palliative and Supportive Care. (In Press).

INDEX